Journey Into Darkness

BY

RONALD SIMPSON, JR.

authorHOUSE®

AuthorHouse™
1663 Liberty Drive, Suite 200
Bloomington, IN 47403
www.authorhouse.com
Phone: 1-800-839-8640

First published by AuthorHouse 11/20/2007

ISBN: 978-1-4343-3575-3 (sc)

Printed in the United States of America
Bloomington, Indiana

This book is printed on acid-free paper.

This is the tale of a 'live and learn' journey while trying to care for an Alzheimer's patient.

Ron Simpson, Jr.

ALZHEIMER'S DISEASE

It is a source of humor for some and a source of pain for others. It is insidious and relentless. Many diseases in this land are just as terrible and if you are associated with someone infected with one of them, that one is number one. I have been associated with heart disease, and cancer, and AIDS, and now, Alzheimer's disease.

One thing I found in each of these cases was that the view on the outside is enormously different from the view on the inside. This is the story of our journey into the darkness that is Alzheimer's disease. Grab a flashlight and follow us.

Prologue:

In the latter part of March, during a family trip to Merritt Island, Florida, Jim Young, Tammy's dad told us that we needed to do something about Carol, Tammy's Mom. He told us of some of the things happening there. He told us that he was unable to handle her anymore. It was more so that he is unwilling to take care of her. Even though she has no drivers' license, he continues to send her to the store. He chose to tell us this on the day before we were to leave for home in Kentucky.

In April, we began to make plans for Jim to bring Carol to us. We checked around. We talked to friends that were familiar with guardianship and nursing homes. For a bit, we actually thought we were prepared.

"Reality paging Ron and Tammy. Is there a Ron or Tammy here? "

Sidebar

Even when your friends warn you about the magnitude of the task before you, you still foolishly think you are ready. There is nothing that can prepare you for the journey you are about to make. Accept that. Make all the preparations you can and still expect the worst. In the movie, "Armageddon", a team of oilrig drillers is chosen to fly into space, drill holes into an asteroid on a collision course with Earth, deposit nuclear bombs, fly off, and detonate them, to destroy the asteroid before it collides with Earth. One of the drillers going to the asteroid asks about the environment on the asteroid. When NASA explains it to him, he sums it up by saying, "You could have just said, "the scariest environment imaginable"". This is not far from that. There are unimaginable pitfalls. There are numerous brick walls. Sources that you think should help will hinder and help will come from places you would not dream.

Accept all the help you can get. It will come at times few and far between. Listen carefully to every bit of information you hear. Glean as much as possible from every source. Thank every person to whom you speak. You may need their help again. Praise efficiency. Ignore ineptness. Keep the goal in mind. There are times you will be angry. Anger serves no ones best interest. Keep a paper trail. Log your phone calls. Write down the details, but do not get lost in them. Take good care of yourself. Have faith.

Saturday, May 8th

The day has arrived. After weeks of talking to Jim Young on the phone and making arrangements, they had begun their journey. At first, they were going to arrive on our doorstep at 6 AM. These plans quickly changed. Then it was going to be 8 AM. Then it was going to be noon. A call around 10AM from a drunken Jim Young in North Carolina put the new arrival time around 3PM. Then, around 5PM, they called to say they were leaving Jim's brother, Uncle Deanie's house in Richmond, KY and on their way here. They arrived at approximately 7PM. A friend from Florida, Mike, had driven them up. Jim and Carol were both intoxicated. Jim stayed long enough to clean out the van, drink a few more beers, and tell us that Carol had $400 in her purse. He and Mike then got in the van and left, telling Carol they were going to the store.

We took Carol with us to the Eleventh Frame Lounge at Southland Bowling Lanes to distract her. We kept her there until close to midnight and then proceeded home. Once we arrived home, Carol was adamant about us taking her home. She thought it was just across town. We explained that Jim had returned to Florida and that she was staying with us. For the next two hours, she stood in the yard or sat on the porch, cursing Jim Young, and demanding that we take her home. During this time, she went from thinking that she was in Florida and Jim was in Kentucky, to thinking that Jim was on the porch talking, to demanding that we drive her home so she could feed her dog. It was 3AM and with the help of an anti-depressant, we got Carol into the house and onto the couch to sleep.

Sunday, May 9th

Shortly after waking, Carol began demanding that we take her back to Florida. We finally placated her by agreeing that if she would see a doctor and the doctor agreed that she was well enough, that we would put her on the Greyhound bus to Florida. This worked, even though she had to be reminded of the agreement from time to time.

She still refuses to accept that Jim dropped her off and went back to Florida. She vacillates from wanting to make sure her furniture is safe from that 'lying Jim Young' to worried that he is bringing in 'two bit whores', to needing to feed her dog, to thinking that her house is just across town.

It is Mother's Day. We had to cancel our plans to go to church this morning because it would not be possible. We cannot take Carol with us. She is still much too agitated. One of us would have to stay with her.

We were going to go to deliver my Mother's Day gift to mom together, but just as we were about to leave, Carol awoke. Tammy stayed home with her while I went to take our best to Mom. This was the tip of the iceberg.

Arguing with Carol is useless. Five minutes after you win the argument, she has forgotten that it took place and rehashes the entire issue. I simply talk to her calmly. As much as I can without compromising key points, I agree with her (some things she does remember). It is harder for Tammy (understandably so). She remembers Carol when she was young and very sharp. Carol was the bookkeeper for a company that did work at Kennedy Space Center. She is very intelligent. It hurts her to see that once thriving intelligence hampered by this disease. She frustrates easily. This is not a judgment, merely an observation.

Monday, May 10

I started the day on the phone, calling Breckenridge (private care facility) and UK Center on Aging, seeking information as to where we should begin. This led to a game of phone tag with referrals and information.

During the morning round of calls, Jim called. We asked him about Carol only having $20 in her purse. He said he did not understand that, but would wire us $100 for some of her expenses.

When asked what happened to her Social Security check, he told us he used it to pay the rent (on a house in which she was not going to live). We also informed him at that time that he was not to do anything with the furniture in the house that belonged to Carol. Carol's father, Odas Oliver, made it. We will have to arrange to get it here once Carol is settled in somewhere.

After many phone calls and much advice, we took Carol to the ER at St. Joe Hospital where they diagnosed her with Stage 3 of Alzheimer's disease. A psychologist from Ridge Behavioral Health was called in and she issued a statement saying that Carol was not able to care for herself, unable to make appropriate decisions, and is a risk to herself and possibly others. St. Joe was going to send her to Eastern State Mental Hospital until it was determined by them that they could not because we were not her legal guardians. St. Joe suggested we take her to Eastern State Mental Hospital ourselves. Eastern State said they could not take her if we brought in. Eastern State said they could take her in if the police brought her in. On the drive home, Carol hit Tammy, so we decided to call the police in. When the police came, they informed us that Eastern State had lied, but that the police could not take Carol in unless they had physical evidence of the assault, or they heard her threaten to harm herself. The officer asked Carol if she was going to hurt herself. She said that she was not intending to harm herself. I have to wonder how many times this tactic works.

The officer then suggested that we take her to University of Kentucky Medical Center for evaluation, since UKMC is linked to the State and St. Joe is not. We called UKMC to confirm this. They let us know they could evaluate her but could not assure us they would keep her. UKMC suggested calling Eastern State Mental Hospital. We called Eastern State and they told us to come there and get a petition and take it to District Court. We did this. Judge Ransdale issued the order. The sheriffs arrived and escorted Carol to Eastern State Mental Hospital for 72-hour involuntary evaluation. That was at 9:30 PM.

Tuesday, May 11

Following the advice of Eastern State Mental Hospital and David Gottfried of the Legal Helpline For Older Kentuckians, Tammy went to the Division of Mental Health to apply for emergency guardianship. The clerk rudely asked why she was applying for emergency guardianship, accused her of trying to get Carols money (she has none), and refused to allow her to file. She told her that she did not believe that Jim Young had 'dropped' Carol off. She accused us of writing the referral from Ridge Behavioral Health ourselves. She stated that she did not believe that Carol was as bad as was reported because if she were so bad, she would not have left her somewhere. When Tammy informed her that Carol was not here because she was at Eastern State Mental Hospital, she asked why we needed an emergency hearing. She told Tammy that she would give us the paperwork for regular guardianship and promised us she would make it take six months.

Upon returning home, with the paperwork for guardianship, we called David Gottfried of LHFOK for advice. David suggested calling Wayne Cook, assistant DA. I left a message with his secretary asking him to return my call. We then called Adult Protective Services and spoke with Mac Colliver. He had no idea why the clerk would have refused to allow us to file. He told us that Wayne Cook was our source of information in this since Mr. Cook will have to present the case to Judge Alexander.

We are wearing out both cell phones and the house phone with all the calling. While Tammy was on the phone with the DR's office about Chelsea, her 13-year-old daughter, and I am on the phone with someone else, my phone rings. I cannot answer immediately, but picked up the message within a minute. It is Lexington Traditional Magnet School. They need us to call back immediately. Chelsea cannot breathe. I call them back as Tammy is putting the inhaler in her purse to take to them. They have already called 911. Tammy arrives at the school (after breaking several land speed records) to find fire trucks and an ambulance waiting. She gives Chella two tokes off the inhaler and brings her home, waving off the offers to take her to the ER. Chella thought the EMT's were cute. Sounds like a typical teenage girl to me.

Tuesday, May 11th Afternoon

Wayne Cook returned my call around 1PM. Once the situation was explained to him, he told me to go to the clerk's office with the paperwork we were given and to ask for the emergency petition as well. He was calling the clerk's office to tell them to give us those papers. He said that he would try to get her hearing on Friday, the 14th. He stated that based on our phone conversation, he felt that the emergency guardianship was warranted. We actually took a breath, finally.

In between running Sierra, Tammy's 15-year-old daughter, to the DR and me picking up Kyle, her 8-year-old son, Tammy made it to the Division of Mental Health to file the petition for emergency guardianship. Both forms had to be filed (as near as we can figure, the second had to be filed in case the emergency is rejected). This is something that we will check. The forms are filed, however, and we have a hearing date for the 18th of May, at 8:30AM. Both forms have to be filed because the emergency guardianship is limited in its scope to the powers imposed by the Judge hearing the petition. There still needs to be a petition for full guardianship in place to pick up where the other leaves off.

Wednesday, May 12th

Already today has started with bumps. The clerk's office called and did not have the addresses for St. Joe Hospital or Ridge Behavioral Health, even though they work with these people all the time in this field. This is just another part of the bureaucratic bull you can run into if you piss off a public servant. The clerk from yesterday was still snippety when Tammy filed the emergency papers. I suppose this is her revenge. Lord, deliver us from small-minded civil servants. We made a few calls and the addresses were called into the clerk's office.

They now have their three ounces of flesh (hard to get a pound of flesh these days, with inflation and such).

We are still fighting with Social Services about the kid's doctor situation. Sierra still is wearing the brace, not knowing if wrist is broken or not. Chelsea is out of school today with her asthma. Her primary care provider now says that they have released her as well and refuses to see her. As you may recall, Lexington Traditional Magnet School called 911 yesterday when Chelsea was having difficulty breathing. She has an inhaler, but is not allowed to have it at school because it is not in the box with the DR's info on it. The school has now decided that she can have it in her purse. I convinced Tammy that she needed to go to physical therapy for her wrist today. She went, but only for me. I am including all of this so that others will understand one very simple and basic concept. The Earth does not stop revolving around the sun just because you have encountered a crisis. The centrality of your life may have shifted, but the rest of it continues as usual. Kids still get sick or hurt. The car still needs an oil change. You still have to jiggle the handle on the toilet when you flush. Somewhere in the middle of all the handle jiggling, temperature taking, and routine maintenance, you still have to find a nursing home, provide info to clerks, take clothes to your mother/ mother-in-law, and fix delightfully nutritious meals.

Here is a word to all you working fathers. Do not think or imply that your wife can take care of all of this because she is a homemaker and has more time. Her day is every bit as full as yours is. When this is all said and done, she will know more about this process than you can imagine. Keep her on your side. She will be your most valuable asset during this time. Buy her a flower. Bring home supper. Anything you can do to make her job easier or to make her smile will make your life much better. Trust me. I am involved in this just like Tammy, but she does more running, makes more phone calls, and carries the greater burden, because this is her Mom. I know in my heart, however, that she would be just as dedicated and just as busy, if it were my Mom.

There is an inner strength you have not tapped. There is courage that you have not used. You have not even begun to feel the real determination yet. Learn to cherish the quiet. Believe me; you will tire of the ringing phone. You will weary of giving the same information to a dozen people in one call, only to be told that it is not something they deal with, but let me transfer you to someone that does. It amazes me that there are some many uncrossed **t's** and undotted **i's** in this world.

Do not lose hope.

Today we will make a trip to Eastern State to see Carol. We will take her some clothes and a pair of sneakers, as she had only one set of clothes and some low-heeled dress shoes going in. Visiting hours are 2-4 PM and 6-8 PM. It will be good to see her, even though it will be difficult. Here is a piece of advice for you. Try to see as much of your loved ones personality as you can, even through the sickness. Do not let your mind disassociate them and relegate them into just a task. Feel the pain; it will become a source of strength. See the humor; it will feed your soul. If you have younger children (we have 3 here, 8, 13, and 15), do not hide this process from them. It is ok to let them see your frustration. Of course, do not take that frustration out on them. Do not snap at them. Do not push them away. You need them now more than ever. Keep their lives as normal as possible, but allow them to observe this process.

It is 9:30 AM. The day has already been long.

Here we are. It is now 11:30 AM, and the phone dialing has begun in earnest. Let's back up just a moment and give a brief explanation. Carol drives in Florida. She has a revoked license. Several times in the past couple years for various reasons, she has been ticketed by local and state police agencies. She missed several court dates and some bench warrants were issued for her for 'failure to appear'. Carol has very little concept of time where days are concerned. This is not so much a condition of the Alzheimer's. Tammy says she has always been a little off in that.

We were in Merritt Island for a week during March. We were awakened on a Friday morning by Carol telling us she that she had to go to court and the SOB Jim Young was gone off somewhere in her van. Therefore, off we go to Titusville, where we learn that she was supposed to be there two days earlier, and another bench warrant has been issued. Tammy talks to the clerks there and gets them to reschedule the court appearance to the 20th of April. We begin the trip home that evening.

Several days prior to the 20th, we call Jim to remind him that Carol has a court appearance. The 20th comes and goes, and Carol does not appear in court. Another bench warrant was issued. On May 1, the sheriff arrives and arrests Carol. Jim posts $300 bond and she was released. All of this is now our problem as well. Alzheimer's patients rarely come without luggage. The Titanic did not have this much luggage and we all know what happened to it.

This morning, we have called every public official in Florida. Ok, not really. They are trying to help us. Justice via long distance, ain't technology grand? (Remember the statement about seeing the humor. This is where that comes in very handy.) After much phone jumping, we found a man that really wanted to help as much as he could. To Josh, at the clerk's office in Melbourne, Florida, we say, Thank you! He gave us valuable information and numbers. One of the things he gave us was the number to Christa, Judge Turner's assistant. The first ten times we called, we got a voice message that said Christa was away from her desk, with no 'leave a message' option. Oddly enough, call number eleven got thru to a voice message that did allow us to leave a number. Tammy left a few messages with case numbers and numbers to call back. We will see how slowly the wheels of justice turn.

Oh yeah, the Rite Aid Pharmacy has the prescription for the Albuterol, for the nebulizer, called in yesterday by the DR's office that claims they released Chelsea two years ago, and has never seen her one time. This is interesting, to say the least. She has had one breathing treatment so far and is breathing better. St. Joe Hospital called and informed us as to the result of Sierra's x-rays. No break! There are still pockets of good news. Family Services has called.

There seems to be movement on the western front. We are just hoping that it is not a bowel movement. Actually, they have assigned the kids to a new primary care provider and now they can be seen, medically. Take your victories wherever you can get them.

We find it somewhat interesting, that, of all the people who were so concerned about Carol on Saturday, none have called to check her status. Do not be surprised when you are doing this all alone. Be grateful and expressive when help does come. Do not be dismayed when it does not.

One more thing; always get the name of the person on the phone.

Tammy wants to have a nervous breakdown, but we cannot seem to find time in our schedule to allow it. Maybe when this is over, we will find time and place for a nice quiet breakdown. Personally, I want a business card sized card that I can hand out before dealing with anyone, family, and friends included. This card will say,

"I am in the middle of a crisis right now.
Please excuse me while I bite your head off.
I will return to myself eventually.
Thank you and have a nice day."

Lunch is over. Was that a three-minute power nap? Life and the ringing phone go on. There is still no word back from Judge Turner's office.

We went to visit Carol at Eastern State. The guard at the gate issued us visitor and parking passes and directed us to the back of the complex. We found the building with no trouble. Once inside, however, the story was different. There was no one to point us in the direction we needed to go. Finally, a woman came into the building that looked like she might know what she was doing (she was carrying a clipboard. I am firmly convinced that you could take over the country if your army carried clipboards instead of guns. Perhaps George W should have been looking for clipboards of mass destruction.). She directed us incorrectly, but caught us in time to rectify her error. We rode an old and slow elevator to the proper floor.

Once out of the elevator, we found the door with its boldly displayed sign. AWOL RISK. The woman who graciously allowed us entrance took our bags of clothes for Carol for inspection.

We visited Carol for a while. She told us she hated that we had to come all that way just to see her. We assured her that it was no trouble. She signed the papers making Tammy her representative payee for her SS check. We told her of the clothes that we brought. She has lost her glasses somewhere. The nurse checked her picture, taken when she got there, and she did not have them on her face, or her head. She told us about her DR, with his jet-black hair (she is sure he colors it), and his fine looks. She told us she has known him for years. Visiting hours were close to over. She walked us to the desk, where we requested something for her headache. We bid her farewell. She again told us she was worried that we had come so far. We told her that we were going to stay close by and that we would see her tomorrow. She was much calmer. We wondered what drugs they have her on.

Chasity, my 21-year-old daughter, her husband Chris, and son Ian came by for a short visit. It was good to see them. My newest grandson now weighs 10 pounds 6 ounces. I finally got Tammy to give him up, held him for a bit, and sang to him.

Evening came. Things were calm. We took the kids to Wal-Mart. Sierra had some money she just had to spend. Tammy and I drove across town to give a CD I had burned to a friend. It was good to laugh with him and to laugh with each other on the drive. We sang together as we drove back to pick up the kids. Once home, Tammy took a bubble bath and then we sat on the couch and watched a movie, almost without interruptions.

I mentioned earlier about how, even though you are in the midst of this crisis, daily living does not go away. You must work to make sure that the positive side of daily living continues as well. You must not let your predicament own you. Do what you must to keep in touch with yourself. Keep this dilemma in its proper place. Yes, there are times that it will spill out of the boundaries. It will flow into your evening meal. It will invade your quality time. Tub water splashed onto the floor is not a terrible thing. You cannot let the water rule the house, however.

Here it is, just after midnight. Another full day of gathering information, making phone calls, making decisions, and chipping away at brick walls waits on the other side of tonight. Tammy has just gone to bed and I am finishing my day with this entry. This is my 'keeping it in perspective'. When this is over (yes, it actually does end) I will look back and read this and re-smile the smiles, re-cry the tears, and wonder how we ever got through it. Purposely, I have segmented this by the days. I know that the only way to get thru this is one day at a time. You will not make one phone call and fix it all. You will not make one trip and be over. You will do each day what you can and take the lessons learned on that day, tuck them in your belt, and run headlong into the next one. Tomorrow, you will be older. Tomorrow, you will be wiser.

Thursday, May 13th

Thursday is Jordan day for Sierra. Jordan is Sierra's boyfriend. Tammy takes Kyle to school, drops Chelsea off at her school, and then drives across town to pick up Jordan at the Dairy Mart close to his house. Sierra is not allowed at Jordan's house by law of his parents. That is a completely different story, which we will not ever touch here. Anyway, Tammy picks up Jordan and takes him to Eastside Vocational School. This allows Sierra and him to see each other for about 20 minutes one morning a week. This is a usual thing. It is part of our routine that we try not to allow this to affect. Granted, if it does, it just does, and we can work other ways for them to see each other.

Sierra has ADHD. It helps to keep her on a regular schedule. This is just part of that effort. We home school her. Has this disrupted her routine? YES. I am sure most of you have heard of ADHD, but do not know how familiar you might be with it. Let me take a minute to tell you a little about Sierra's case. She does not take Ritalin or other drugs for it. They turn her into a zombie. She does take a natural alternative. The problem with her is more the ADD than the HD part. She has trouble staying on task. When we are teaching her, any interruption will practically erase what she has learned. Learning is a process of stacking blocks. When the process is interrupted in her, she loses most of the blocks. This has scattered blocks all over the house. Tammy calls it 'tornado day at Romper Room'.

While Tammy was at PT, (Sierra was with her. No time between running here to there), Randy Moeler, a social worker working with Carol, called. He asked about Jim being an alcoholic. I told him he was not, but that he was a drunk at times. He asked about Mary Oliver (although he did not know her name). Carol talked to him about that she would be willing to go into the nursing home where her mother is staying. He asked about her sources of income. I told him about her Social Security for $618 and whatever miniscule money she and Jim might raise with the scrap metal business. I gave him Tammy's cell phone number.

Once she returned, Tammy managed to fix a cup of coffee and some buttered toast, before she began with phone calls. She got through to Christa at Judge Turner's office in Florida. She is to fax the papers from the DR evaluation and the guardianship papers, when we get them. Tammy takes this accomplishment as a victory. It is just after 11 o'clock.

We made it all the way until 12:30 PM before the next crisis, albeit a small one. The nurse at Lexington Traditional Magnet School called to tell us that Chelsea had to use her inhaler and she thinks that there may be the beginnings of bronchitis. She says that Chelsea needs to see her DR in the next 12 to 14 hours. She thought Chella would be okay to stay at school, but was going to take her temperature and call us back if she felt it necessary for her to come home. Tammy calls Kentucky Clinic North, the kid's new primary care provider, to schedule an appointment. They tell us they can see her next Thursday. This will not work, we explain. Upon hearing the circumstances for the need to be seen, April suggests that we take Chella to the Urgent Treatment Center on Custer Dr.

Problem number One: Chelsea and the kids have just been assigned to KCN as their primary care provider. Their medical card still has their previous provider listed (the one that claims they discharged them two years ago). UTC would call them to get a referral. They will not provide one. We asked if KCN could provide the referral over the phone.

Problem number two: Since the kids were just assigned, KCN does not have them in their system yet. Therefore, they cannot refer them over the phone.

Solution: KCN suggests that we take Chella to the ER. This is more costly to the system and generally much slower. However, Chelsea needs to be seen. So, after school today (the nurse has not called), she will be going to some ER. Ah, life in the slow lane.

Tammy is pissed. She had scheduled a small nervous breakdown for later this afternoon, barring any unforeseen higher-ranking catastrophe. I am thinking that this qualifies and will force cancellation of said breakdown. She is checking the schedule for a more appropriate time.

Calls to nursing homes begin in earnest. This is a delightful process where you explain the private details of your life to hundreds of individuals that will tell you that you need to speak to someone else. Refine your beginning story to the most basic details until you find that one individual that has the answers.

"I am looking for placement of my mother. She has Alzheimer's disease. She has Medicare/Medicaid."

You will be asked questions about the patient's ability to dress, eat, take medicine, go to the bathroom, and so forth, depending on the care level available at each facility.

Susan Marvin, at Royal Manor Nursing Home, was very helpful. She did not have any beds available this week, but might have one ready on Monday. She informed us that Medicare would take care of 100% of the first twenty-one days if she were coming from a hospital. After day twenty-two and until day one hundred, Medicare pays part and supplemental insurance, such as Medicaid, pays the rest. For long-term care, over one hundred days, Medicaid will be the primary payer and her Social Security check, minus forty dollars a month for personal care, pays the rest.

Tammy has moved her operation to the porch where she can smoke a cigarette. Armed with the phone book, pen, paper, and a wealth of questions, she tackles this phase. Welcome to 'learn as you go'.

Melissa Morris, with Rose Manor, says they have no beds, but are adding Carol to the waiting list. She did the assessment over the phone and told us that they would accept her if a bed became available.

Pinewood Place, listed in the yellow pages under nursing homes, is not a nursing home. They are just an apartment complex.

Sherry, the assistant administrator for the Lexington Center for Health and Rehabilitation, says they have no beds. They placed Carol on their waiting list as well. Our friend, Jana, works for this nursing facility.

We have discovered that we do not really need a nursing home, per say. What we really need are 'personal care beds'.

Rebecca, the assistant admissions coordinator for Rose Terrace says that they do have beds. She did the assessment over the phone and is giving the information to Jennifer, the admissions coordinator. They will contact Eastern State Mental Hospital and get the information they need. Tammy has to contact them tomorrow.

Tammy then called Homestead Nursing home. She volunteered there during the summers from when she was thirteen until she was sixteen. The admissions coordinator, Janet McRobert, said that they did have beds. Tammy is to call Eastern State and have them fax the info to them.

There are terms that we have learned, such as personal care, nursing care, and invalid care. We have also learned the criteria for each of these. Personal care is defined as assisted living care for individuals deficient in two or more areas of personal care. These include but are not limited to feeding, dressing, incontinence, and grooming. Nursing home care is for individuals that meet the above criteria but also have medical care issues that require registered nursing care. Invalid care is someone that requires round the clock care and is unable to do anything for themselves.

In addition, women's beds are harder to find. We figure this is because on the longer life expectancy for women.

Here is one more piece of advice. Take care of yourself. Tammy and I take vitamin supplements. This is no time to let your own health suffer. You need to be strong during this ordeal.

Oh yeah, the toilet is broken. I will be going to some hardware store and getting a replacement 'fluidmaster' flow valve. Life goes on. Also in the midst of all of this, we are trying to help Dad rent the apartment above us. We have been painting, doing electrical work, drywall ceiling repair, and plumbing. The ad goes into the paper today with Dads number being the primary contact and mine in the ad as well. Therefore, while we are picking up children from school, visiting Carol, and taking Chella to the ER, we have to pick up toilet repair parts.

Somewhere in the middle of all of this, you will say these words, "I cannot do this". It will not be true and you really will not mean it. You just have to say it to get it out of the way.

Tammy picked Kyle up from school and then off she went again. Kyle and I went to Bobby and Kathy's house to help Bobby with the electric work on his new playhouse. Kathy and Bobby are my sister and brother-in-law. He has built a new shed for his work area. It is about sixteen feet by eight feet. We put in six outlets, four lights, and two switches. I was already in the middle of helping when this whole situation broke open. Right at the start of it, while I was delivering my Mom's Day gift, Kathy called to talk to Mom. I answered the phone. She tells me that Bobby has cut off the tip of his finger because he has no help. He thinks I just do not want to help him. Therefore, I talk to her and Bobby and give them the briefest scenario I could about why I have been, and will continue to be, busy. Bobby had a DR appt. today and was home early. I told him it would be easier if we worked early, since evenings were mostly taken with kid activities.

My baby sister, Patty got there a while after I did. She was happy to see me, as I was to see her. While Bobby went to Lowe's to get more supplies, I came into the house and chatted with Patty. I told her about the Carol ordeal (Please do not misunderstand the use of the word 'ordeal'. Erase the negative connotation. It is just a nearly overwhelming, totally unprepared for, situation.).

Kyle learned how to use T-5 wire strippers. He learned how to cut the wire, strip the insulation, bend the hook, and squeeze it closed. We got the feed into the house and hooked it up. All of the receptacles are now working. I still have to install the switches and mount two of the lights, but that is tomorrow's project.

I called Tammy. She was at Rite Aid, dropping off a prescription and then she was on her way home to fix supper. Kyle and I loaded up our tools. Supper was on the horizon. On the way home, we stopped at Lowe's and got the washer to fix the toilet. Kyle played 'run and hide and sneak up on Ron' throughout the entire trip inside. We had fun.

Supper was great. Afterwards, Tammy and the girls went to see Carol. Eastern State has her on medication for Alzheimer's disease. While she is still scattered, she is much calmer. She realizes that she is in Kentucky. She specifically asked Tammy if we were looking for a place for her to live, here in Kentucky. Tammy told her that we were, and told her what kind of place.

Tammy says she is going to start recording what she tells Carol, so that, when she asks the same question for the umpteenth time, she can save her vocal cords and just play the recording. Perhaps she can listen to it at night and absorb the information subliminally in her sleep.

This thing invades our conversations. If not watched, it can completely monopolize the moment. While we do need to talk about it, we need to keep other conversations alive. This proves to be difficult at times, with friends and family asking how it is going.

It is 11:46 PM. Kyle is sleeping. Chelsea is sleeping and coughing. Sierra is involved in her conversation with Jordan. Tammy has just gone to bed. The light is on, so I am sure she is reading. Once again, I am winding down the day and getting this out of my mind. Saving it here seems to help clear it out of my head. It has not marched into my dreams yet.

Friday, May 14th

Today did not start out good. We overslept. It was only forty-five minutes, but that is plenty when you are on a tight schedule. This morning was supposed to go something like this: seven AM, Wake up and get the kids up and begin getting them ready for school; 7:45, out the door to drop the kids off at their respective schools and then directly to Physical Therapy (early). After PT, a fast trip to the Social Security office to check on or apply for Medicaid for Carol. This would happen before the office got full. It is a full house on Fridays.

Needless to say, that did not happen. It was after 8AM before Tammy got out the door. She was going to PT after the kid drops, still a bit early. With any luck at all, she might get to Social Security before the crowd. There are still calls to be made to various nursing homes. We still have to make sure that Carol will be taken care of until the hearing. Then, a smooth move into the right nursing facility would be ideal. We have learned not to expect the ideal. Somewhere between the ideal and a raging disaster is usually where it ends up. Sometimes it goes from one end of the spectrum to the other instantly. This is like building a house of cards. One wrong move and it all might tumble down. All the preparations in the world are still resting on one 'iffy' decision that is out of our hands.

It is difficult to explain, but you have to be careful not to get too emotionally detached. You do have to have some emotional detachment when dealing with parts of this. There are legal matters that are not points of passion. There are decisions that have to be made based solely on the merits of that decision alone. There are waiting periods that can drive you crazy. To you, this it the most important thing you are working on. To many of the people that you are dealing with, it is just another part of their everyday job. The drive behind you is not the same as the drive behind them. Your passionate pushing can come across as accusing them of not doing their job. So, deal with the slow parts of the process as well as you can. Learn to trust the eventual. Yes, I actually do know that it is easier said than done.

Tammy marvels at my patience, not only in this, but in other things as well. That is just who I am. That is not to say there are times that I am not patient. I am just patient until I am not patient. A very good friend, and then Assistant Pastor of the church to which I belonged when living in Massillon, Ohio, told me once, that trials would make you bitter or better. This, like the rest of the trials in my life will do that. I am striving for the better side. Bitterness is a seed. Once planted, it will grow and taint every other part of your life. Tammy says that she is not bitter. She is just sour, like a pickle. She does not have the energy to be bitter, she says. Sour is the best she can do at the moment.

It is 10:25 AM and Tammy has returned. She has the Chella with her. It seems that her inhaler was nearly empty and this is not time to be at school with a nearly empty inhaler. She says they broke her in PT today. They made her scrub. This is doing a scrubbing motion on a piece of wood. They could have at least given her a dirty pot to scrub. She told the therapist that she could do scrubbing at home. Her grip strength in her right hand has increased from five pounds to ten pounds. In her left hand, it is seventy-five pounds. She still has a ways to go. She has not made it to the Social Security office yet.

Chelsea asked about the journal and how far along it was. I told her I was on page thirty-nine. She wanted to know how long it was going to be. As long as it will be is as long as it will be, was the only answer I could give her. She says she is still trying to decide if this is a drama or a comedy. Tammy says it is a 'dramedy'. Yes, just as I suspected. That one frightened the automatic spellchecker. Several times throughout this, we will remind you of how important it is to keep your sense of humor. This is one of those times. It is not being unfaithful to the seriousness of the situation to find humor here as well.

Tammy is hungry, so, she fixed some prepackaged scrambled eggs, taters, and sausage. She added extra scrambled eggs and some cheese. We both cook. Finding prepackaged foods in the fridge is rare, but we are trying to help a friend that works for Schwan's. It has paid off during this time.

The evil one is up. What else is there to call a bi-polar ADHD hormonal 15-year-old girl? She has been enjoying her school break. All she has had to deal with this week are her spelling words. The test is today as usual.

Someone once asked me how I spent my spare time. My reply: "Spare time is an illusion. It doesn't really exist, but if I move my hands fast enough you will swear that you actually saw it." We have borrowed time from home schooling. We have borrowed time from sleeping. We have borrowed time from reading and playing games. We already were not big TV watchers, so we could not borrow from that.

Connie Smith at Sayre Christian Village returned our call. She informed us that there are no assisted living facilities in the state of Kentucky that are not private pay. If you want to, or need to, use insurance, you have to go to a personal care facility, even if the patient does not require personal care. She said that incontinence is always a good way to get someone into a personal care facility. It is a very thin line between personal care and full time nursing care. Full time nursing care is substantially higher. It requires more insurance or higher self pay. The only way full time nursing care facilities will accept Medicare/Medicaid/Social Security is if the patient has a life threatening illness. Documentation is the key. Gather every record that you can. Talk to every doctor they have seen. Save every piece of paper that looks remotely related. Keep bank records to show financial responsibility. You are going to have to convince several people in important positions that this person you love can no longer take care of themselves. Keep in mind; you are not degrading them. You are going through a process to insure that they are cared for properly. I wish Tammy and I could retire and provide her mother the care she needs. That is not going to be a possibility. To insure that this happens, we have to play with their ball, run their bases, and play by their rules. Sometimes, it sucks. Heck, most of the time, it sucks.

Tammy and the girls visited Carol this afternoon for the 2 until 4 visitation. I stayed home with Kyle. He is too young to visit. When Tammy returned, she had the papers from the initial examination by Randy Moeler and E. Cifuentes, M.D. Carol told them that she moved from Kennedy Space Center, which is in Kentucky. She reports that she has no children. She says she has been divorced for six months. She and Jim divorced nineteen years ago in 1985. The report states that she is very confused disorganized in her speech and extremely tangential. Grab your medical terminology dictionary. Tammy says that Carol now believes the hospital is in Florida and we have moved there as well. Imagine the effect of reading this report, if it were talking about your mother or father. This is not going to be an easy task, even though it is the right thing to do.

Imagine how Carol must feel. There are thoughts, jumping in and out of her mind, which she is trying desperately to bond. She is trying to make sense of the chaos in her head. She is filling in the gaps. There is a strange segmental logic here. She cannot see the entire picture anymore. She sees bits and pieces without timeframe. She is inside there somewhere, fighting to maintain her cohesiveness. It is akin to walking into a town to which you have never been, and trying to find your house there.

Do not see this as her weakness. This takes monumental strength to even try to make it sensible. She is fighting a battle with weapons that only scarcely work. For brief moments at various times, she wins, until the pool of confusion overwhelms her again.

Saturday, May 15th

There are no offices to call. There are no hospitals to contact. There are no Government programs to follow up. This is actually a free day. Well, it is a relatively free day. Sierra had a meeting at work at 10AM and she has to be back at work at 6PM. I need to go the Kathy and Bobby's to finish the electric work. Also, Gretchen, a friend talked to me online this morning. She is still hurting from the death of her father some weeks ago. Tammy and I are going to get up with her this evening sometime.

It is seventeen minutes past one o'clock in the afternoon. There was supposed to be someone here at one to view the apartment upstairs. She has not made it yet and has not called. I talked with a friend about the apartment. He might be interested. He has two small boys around Kyle's age. That would be a welcome break. Imagine Kyle having someone to play with and not asking us a hundred questions a day. Do not get me wrong. I love Kyle. Usually I will answer his questions, but there are days when he asks excessively many questions and questions that do not matter. He asked me, a day, or so ago, if he killed someone accidentally, is that a sin? I asked him if he planned to kill anyone accidentally. He does ask some interesting questions. It is intriguing to see the way his mind works. Those things he cannot figure out, he creates working solutions. The solution may only work in Kyle-realm, but it works.

He has a very active fantasy imagination. He and I are super hero's that work for a top-secret organization that is responsible for all life on planet Earth. This morning, he told me that he quit his job. He is no longer going to moonlight as a super hero. This is going to cause a gap in the schedule, as I am on vacation during this time as well. I am sure, however, that someone will step into the gap. After all, that is what super hero's do.

Reading this as I write it, he has decided that he wants his old job back. He called the 'boss' and reapplied. Of course, he was rehired on the spot. Sleep easy. The world is safe once more.

How nice it would be if all the problems we have could be solved as easy as an imaginary phone call on a toy cell phone.

Kyle has borrowed my cell phone to call his dad in Florida. I think both are coming to terms with the fact that Kyle can love two different men as 'Dad'. Kyle is accepting it faster than Ronnie is.

Between Tammy and myself, there are seven children and four grandchildren. My daughters love Tammy. I have three, ages 24, 20, and 16. The oldest two are married, but the oldest, Audrey, and her hubby, Adam, are filing for divorce. They have three children.

Chasity, my middle daughter, just had a son on the Third of March. Heather, my baby, is 16 and lives with her Mom in Nicholasville. We do not see each other nearly as often as I would like, but we talk on the phone often, and send Emails back and forth almost daily. I talk to her online in Instant Messages also.

Tammy's oldest, Chris, lives in Florida with his dad. He will be 18 in July. Sierra, 15, Chelsea, 13, and Kyle, 8, live here with us. It is one big happy family for the most part. Although, the Morgan clan was a little intimidated at the annual Christmas dinner just past, as they were the newcomers in a crowd of fifty. It worked out okay. No one was bitten.

I come from a very close-knit family. My granny is eighty-nine and still very active. Dad is seventy-three and Mom is sixty-nine. Dad is a retired Pastor and retired electrician. He still very actively preaches. Practically every Tuesday night, he preaches at a house meeting in Berea. Mom still leads songs at the church they now attend. Both are very active. This left me with no practical experience in dealing with Alzheimer's disease. Here we are, suddenly thrust into the middle of a strange town and trying to find our house.

It is almost two o'clock here. I am off to do some electrical work.

It is four o'clock and I am back at home after finishing Bobby's shed. Just before we left, Kyle brought in the mail. We got the information that I requested from the Alzheimer's organization. We were talking about it just this morning. Tammy made a joke, saying, "Maybe they forgot to send it." Tammy went through the papers and determined that her mom is actually in the second stage of Alzheimer's, based on her overall symptoms. They also sent some pamphlets with the papers. They are, "Responding to persons with Alzheimer's disease," "Structuring the day at home," "Overcoming challenges and adapting to the needs persons with Alzheimer's disease," and "Interacting with persons with Alzheimer's disease". In the short time that I have taken to scan them, I can see that they will be helpful.

Tammy is going to visit Carol while I take Sierra to work and pick Kyle up from Kathy's house. Tammy and Kyle went with me to work there. Their grandson, Austin, was there. Kyle stayed to play with him. Tammy is making fudge, which is one of her comfort foods. She just came in with offers of chocolaty kisses. I accepted. Chelsea and Sierra are still sleeping. They stayed up until after 4AM this morning. Chella cleaned the house a bit and fixed a pot of coffee for her mom. She is sprawled out in the waterbed. Sierra is sleeping in her bed. It is quiet. It is scary, because it feels so good. It is so difficult to obtain and so easily broken.

It has been a difficult day for Tammy. She visited Carol today. Carol was more confused than during previous visits. What we considered a godsend, the un-busy-ness of today, is working against her. She has more time to think about the situation on emotional terms. She is fully aware that this will work out. She knows in her head, and in her heart, that Carol will be taken care of. This gives her more time to think about the Carol she has known and the Carol of today. That is a thought process completely different from the one we have been focused on for days. There is also the consideration of the emotional turmoil yet ahead.

Tammy is a thinker. Her mind works all the time. She cannot help it. An old preacher friend of mine says, of thoughts, "you can't stop a bird from flying over your head, but you don't have to let him make a nest in your hair". Tammy has not learned that trick. She cannot stop the thoughts that enter her head. She entertains them to her own pain. As much as I wish I could, I cannot take all of that away from her.

Sunday, May 16th

Another day with no government calls to make. This is a good thing. There are also no nursing homes to call. We took advantage of the day and did some needful things around here. Tammy still struggles with the emotional part. She has refused to allow Jim Young to know anything about Carol other than that fact that she is OK. As far as he knows, and as far as he will know, she is here at the house with us.

We visited her this afternoon. It was a good visit. She is anxious about getting out. They have told her that we are looking for a place her. She goes in and out, about where she is, exactly. Regardless of where she thinks she is, she still thinks that Jim is nearby. She calls him the 'great and mighty asshole.' She still worries about her furniture and her dog.

After our visit, Tammy and I went to the movies. We thought we might actually get some peace. We were not even close to being right. Chelsea called twice. Sierra called us twice. Jim called us once. I answered Sierra's call. She was home from work. Tammy called Jim after the movie was over. He wanted to know what was going on. He was surprised that we were able to go to the movie. We take our peace where we can find it. It is fleeting at best.

We have discovered that Alzheimer's is not a disease of one. It is a family disease. The ironic thing about it is that we have chosen to accept it. Carol did not choose to have it. Jim chose to put it somewhere else. We accept that we cannot handle this alone, but we have accepted the part that is ours. This is not about our 'nobility'. This is just us doing what we know in our hearts is the right thing.

Monday, May 17th

Today started normally. The clock alarm sounded just like it did before. It was just as lacking in mercy as it ever was. Tammy dropped the kids off at school and went to physical therapy. She came back a little less broken than previous visits. She hates the scrub brush. She can tell you about it sometime.

Tammy stretched out on the couch with her book, not as much to read, as to have a reason to lie down. Jennifer, with Rose Manor, called to tell us they had one bed and one person in front of Carol on the list. If this person turns down the bed, Carol can get it. Tammy has to return a call to Royal Manor tomorrow. Both are located in Nicholasville. Interestingly, I discovered today that the Apostolic Lighthouse Church holds services at Royal Manor. This is where my parents attend and the minister, that married Tammy and I, pastors.

Tammy returned to the couch and her book, which she proceeded to read, through closed eyes. Sierra watched a movie about the death penalty and wrote a short essay on her feelings about said penalty and why she feels as she does.

When time came, Tammy went to get Kyle from school. She brought him home and took Sierra with her to visit Carol. I picked Chelsea up from school. When Tammy came home from her visit, she was calmly upset. She explained that Carol had left Jim several times before. In each of those, Jim Young was the worst example of manhood ever born for the first week or so. After that, she would begin to defend his actions. It seems that even the Alzheimer's did not change this.

Carol has an idea that Tammy is going to control her visitors. I do not know if this is a part of her delusion or not. It may be something that her social worker or court appointed attorney told her. We do not even know yet if she has even met her attorney. She would not see that as something that is important enough to tell us. Tomorrow is the big day. The guardianship hearing is tomorrow at 8:30 AM.

Tuesday, May 18th

This morning began a little bit more rushed than usual. The court hearing was at 8:30AM. Chelsea is usually dropped off at school this time. Therefore, the kids get early drop offs and we are headed to Eastern State Mental Hospital for the hearing.

The hearing, as it turns out, was a formality, for the most part. Carol's court appointed attorney, Stacy, recommended that we be granted guardianship. She felt that was in Carol's best interest. Wayne Cook also recommended that Tammy be granted guardianship. Judge Alexander signed the order giving her the right to make medical decisions, choose Carol's living arrangements, to apply for Medicaid for her, and to handle her financial affairs. The papers will be ready at court this afternoon after one o'clock. Once we have them, we can apply for Carol's Medicaid.

There was an unexpected twist. We discovered while we were there that they had also set a preliminary hearing for committal to Eastern State Mental Hospital. This is not what we want. If she is committed to Eastern State, we will have trouble getting her into a nursing facility. While they have no problem accepting her as an Alzheimer's patient, they would have problems if she were labeled as a mental patient. We talked to Carol's attorney, Stacy Turner. She was unaware of these proceedings. The final hearing was set for one week from today. If we find a placement before then, we can move her directly into that home. Otherwise, we will fight to get her released into our custody and take her home.

Despite this, it is still a victorious day. We are closer to taking care of Carol. In all of this, however, there is a deep feeling of defeat. The fact that we had to do any of this is hard enough. Every time there is another step, it reminds us of every painful detail. Every victory is tainted. Every step forward is laced with pain. We keep reminding ourselves that we are doing the right thing.

It is 4PM. Tammy is happy. She has accomplished much. She returned the call to Jennifer at Rose terrace. She was out for the day.

Wednesday, May 19th

We are baby-sitting Ian today and tomorrow. Jordan Thursday has moved to Wednesday. Tammy took Ian with her on her travels. After kids and Jordan, she went to PT. The staff there thought he was the cutest kid, and he is.

Tammy had not been home very long before Jennifer returned her call. There is a snag. Carol only qualifies for personal care and Medicare does not pay the first twenty-one days. The solution, according to Jennifer, is to bring Carol home and wait until the third of the month when she receives her SS check. They will take her then if we sign the check over to them. They will apply for the Medicaid supplement for her. We are also keeping other nursing home options open. We are to check with Sherry at Lexington Center for Health and Rehab close to the end of the week.

We will request that Carol come home with us at the committal hearing. She does belong in a nursing care facility. She does not belong in a mental institute. Alzheimer's is a disease, not a mental illness. Some people that you encounter, even in the mental health field, will not make this distinction.

Tammy visited Carol today during the later visiting times. She says that it made all the difference in the world. The other patients were much more active than usual. One patient came to where they were sitting. When she finished talking and walked away, Carol turned to Tammy and said, "Get me out of here".

This is the waiting time. We have to accept everyone's schedule. I am convinced that the wheels will never really turn as quickly as we want. We just hope that those wheels are indeed turning.

Tonight around midnight, before going to bed, we checked the messages on the phone one more time. There were several messages about the apartment upstairs. There was one message from Randy Moeler and one from the division of Mental Health for Fayette Co. The call from DMH was concerning the Doctor and Psychiatrist that were listed as diagnosing Carol. We will return those calls in the morning.

Thursday, May 20th

The phone ringing at 6:55AM woke us this morning. It was Ronnie; Tammy's ex, wanting to talk to Kyle, who was still sleeping. I asked him to call back in five minutes and we would wake Kyle. Tammy woke Kyle and Chella and came back to snuggle for another minute. Kyle yelled into the room that someone was at the door. We told him that it was Chasity and to let her in. She was bringing Ian. We chatted briefly and she was off to work. Forty-five minutes later Tammy was out the door to take kids to school. She calls this 'Tammy's Taxi Time'.

At some point in the morning, we begin returning calls. Mine go quickly. I deliver information with the best of them. Tammy then called Randy Moeler. Randy is the social worker at ESMH. She talked to him about the commitment hearing. He told us that Carol could be released to us, when we were prepared to take her. The best-case scenario would be to release her directly to a nursing home. That way there would be as little changes as possible. This would help her adjustment. She could adjust to the move to the nursing facility better than she could adjust to moving here and then to a nursing home. Randy expressed concerns about our ability to care for her. Tammy told him that she was a mental health technician. Her job entails working with mentally handicapped adults. The behaviors of her clients are not all that different from Alzheimer's patients. She takes care of the personal care needs of her clients. She is licensed in CPR and like saving by the American Red Cross. Tammy also dispenses medications to her clients. This allayed some of Randy's concerns.

He suggested that we might want to bring her home for a night to see how it goes. That would be an overnight visit. We discussed this and decided that it would not be a good idea. We feel it would confuse her. Add to this, that she would be agitated about going back to the hospital and it could be perceived by her doctors that she is not ready for home care. We already know that we can care for her. We did it before we had to have her involuntarily evaluated. Randy said he would send home a med pack when we do bring her home. He offered a prescription for Xanax, for either Carol or Tammy. Carol is on the Alzheimer's med and Paxil, a mild antipsychotic drug.

Tammy also addressed the call we received for DMH. Randy said that he would see what he could do about appeasing them.

Next was the call to Division of Mental Health and our favorite clerk. Laura said that the original psychologist was not sufficient for the courts needs. Dr. Carter, the ER physician, offered his help, but would not be allowed because he only saw her in the ER. Tammy explained that Dr. Hawthorne at Eastern State Mental Hospital is a licensed Psychiatrist and therefore a licensed MD as well. Amazingly, Laura was not aware of this. Tammy is going to call Mac Colliver at Adult Protective Services and inquire as to whether they can provide her with a social worker in case Randy was unable to help. Randy's concern was in his training. He is not trained to work with Alzheimer's patients. Carol is his first. What a great way to start.

Between calls, Tammy spoils Ian as much as possible.

The next call was Mac Colliver. He said that the court would petition Adult Protective Services for a social worker. He also said that Laura is just blowing smoke and giving us a hard time. When we get her placed into a nursing home, the doctor there will be the one on record that fills out the papers. Since the hearing is not until July, we have a little bit of time.

He agrees that Carol does not to be committed to Eastern State Mental Hospital. For her own well being and safety, she needs to be home with us until we get her placed. Part of the problem with this is the inability to reach Dr. Hawthorne. It is a thin line. We want what is best for Carol. We agree that she does not need to be committed to Eastern State Mental Hospital. We agree that she does need to be in a nursing facility. It now appears that we will not be able to get her into any facility until after the third of June, when her SS check arrives.

Mac was able to answer questions and address concerns that will make the process easier. Still yet, there are many decisions to be made. There are questions that have not been asked. There are questions that we do not even know to ask. This has more intensity than any class I have ever taken, and the final test holds much more severe consequences than a low grade. Decisions here will affect the rest of our lives and Carol's life as well. How do you do the best, when you are just beginning to see the best as a variable? Every decision has the potential to undo previous decisions. This is becoming more fluid and less static as it progresses. There are no 'cut and dry' answers. Perhaps, the best that we can do is learning the right questions.

Life outside Alzheimer's continues. Cleaning up clutter and pricing it for a yard sale is the next job. We still have to travel to mom's house and pick up more clutter to get rid of. Eventually, the kids will be out of school for the day and Sierra will need a ride to work. The phone still rings with apartment seekers. We still wait. This ordeal weaves its way into the fabric of the rest of your life.

Friday, May 21st

There is almost a feeling of normalcy here. We know that there are still things to do. There are still calls to make. You do not really forget it. You can, however, sometimes let slip to the back of your mind for a few minutes. When you slow down, you can still feel it. It does not go away. Some days, it is easy to keep in below the other things that have to be done. Other days, it just takes over.

The weather is too iffy for the yard sale today. It looks like tomorrow is going to be sale day. There is a thirty percent probability of thunderstorms today. The last couple of days have been filled with sporadic storms. Some have been pretty heavy. Some have been sprinkles.

We hope to find out more about Carol's release today. Tammy left a note for Dr. Hawthorne to set up a time to discuss this with him. Randy has been very accessible. Dr. Hawthorne has not been. She will call him this morning as leaving a note seems ineffectual. She also has to call Judge Turner's office to find out the disposition of Carol's court case. There are always calls to make, it seems. There is always someone that needs some piece of information or another number, or needs to be reminded of something that has been sent twenty-seven times. It can be frustrating at times. You can get fed up. You have to learn to vent to someone other than those that can speed up or slow down the process. At work, we have a saying. "Don't poke the bear. Feed the bear." Take good care of those that have the ability to take good care of you.

Jim called this morning. It turns out that Carol is his representative payee for his SS check. We are wondering how the recently put in change of address for Carol will affect that. Jim says that she is not his rep. payee, but according to the Social Security office, she is. He says that he needs something that says she is in a nursing home. He may or may not get it. Tammy is in a mood. Hey, it happens! It will happen to you too. One day, you will be walking along, and 'BAM', you are in a mood.

12:30 PM

Tammy has just returned from the doctor's office. She did not come home with any good news. First, Dr. Einbecker, the hand specialist recommended by workers Comp, has decided that the surgery he did has caused permanent nerve damage. This pain is now to be a part of her life. He told her that she would never gain full mobility. He has not released her to go back to work. This is not good news.

While at the doctor's office, Eastern State Mental Hospital called to tell her that Carol had been moved into their Alzheimer's unit. Melissa Pierce called to introduce herself as Carol's new social worker. They now say the Dr. Hawthorne feels that she needs to be committed their hospital. Hawthorne says that with her history, no nursing home will take her. This is not the case with any of the nursing homes that we have contacted. We have apprised all of them of her condition and history and all have expressed their willingness to have her as a resident. It looks like we might be in for a fight, come court time. We are not going to lie down and take this one. We will be loaded for bear. We will not allow the state to take away what we have fought so hard to get.

1:30 PM

Melissa is calling. Tammy is discussing her mother's case with her. This may come down to our ability to care for her. Tammy is a licensed mental health technician. She is qualified to dispense medicine. Melissa said that her hands were tied. She did give Tammy the number to the Director of Eastern State, who can override Dr. Hawthorne. We do not know how often that happens, but we are going to do our best to see that this is one of those times. Tammy called and left a message with the director.

We are going to get a job description from ARC. We are going to get statements from the nursing homes that have accepted her.

Evening visitation

We went to see Carol at the Gragg Building. This is the Alzheimer's ward at Eastern State. We visited for a bit and then discussed with the attendants about how we would go about removing Carol AMA (Against Medical Advice). We were told that the only way we could do that was with a doctor's permission. This seemed odd, since we wanted to do it against the doctor's opinion. The charge nurse, Maryann, on the floor did not care much for the fact that we were frustrated. She accused us of being loud and irate and upsetting the patients. We were not loud or irate, nor were any of the patients paying us any mind. Tammy asked to talk to the doctor on call. After asking the fifth time, the charge nurse finally called. The doctor came and looked over the charts. Then we went to a conference room to discuss this. She told us that she had not seen Carol and her hands were tied. The only doctor that could release Carol was Dr. Hawthorne. She explained that since he had initiated a legal petition, only he could stop the process.

She was helpful in several ways. She readily accepted that the mental health process was not user friendly. She was delighted by our concern and efforts and told us that we were not the normal. Most of the patients had no one to look out for them. Most were literally wards of the state. She thought that we would have no trouble getting Carol released to us, because of our efforts at placing her into a nursing home and Tammy's experience working with mental patients. She told us that she would notate on the chart that we had visited and of our intent to care for her ourselves. She also was going to note our efforts to get her into a nursing facility.

We went back the desk to check on Carol and her clothes. One of the attendants took us to her room to check on her clothes. He first took us to the wrong room, which when it was opened, overwhelmed us with the stench of urine. He then took us to the right room. Her clothes were there.

We took Carol outside to explain to her that she would not be going home tonight. She was distraught. She hates where she is. She cried at the idea of staying there for four more nights. She told us that they were crazy there. It was very difficult to leave her. The entire place was dirty. We understand the problem with patients that are incontinent. There will be some smell. This was above that. This was an unkempt odor. We watched the staff interact with the patients. There was a very condescending attitude there. The patients were handled without respect. This is an intolerable situation.

At one point while driving home, I looked at Tammy. She was clenching her fist to white knuckles. There were tears streaming down her face. The emotion has broken through the facade. At home, I asked her if she trusted me. She told me that was the dumbest question she had heard. She trusted me completely. I held her and told her that it was going to be ok.

According to what we were told, Dr. Hawthorne's concerns were that no nursing facility would take Carol and we were not able care for her. We will erase those concerns in the eyes of the court with statements from nursing homes, which have accepted her and put her on their waiting list. As to his concern about us being able to care for her in the interim, Tammy is trained to do just that. Had this pompous ass ever bothered to return our calls, or discuss Carol with us, he would already know this. This will reduce his argument to one of medical opinion. We will ask that another doctor, not associated in any way with Eastern State Mental Hospital or Dr. Hawthorne, examine her.

It is slightly comforting that the on call doctor thinks that we will have no problem getting her released into our custody. There is one thing, however, that we have discovered in all of this. Nothing is sure until it is signed. As hard as we try, as diligently as we fight, as convinced in our hearts as we are, it still is in the hands of someone that does not know Carol or us. We will have the short time of a committal hearing to convince a judge that we are good and capable people. We will be arguing against a disillusioned mental health professional. We will be arguing against his purported facts. We will have us. We will have our love for Carol. We will have right on our side, but right does not always prevail. We are trusting in right and the prayers of our friends and family.

From the outside looking in, this seems like it should be cut and dry. Inside, it is overwhelming. The only way to take it is one day at a time and that is quite difficult in itself. There are days when it seems like it will fly. Then there are other days, and many more like it, when it seems impossible and unbearable. Today is not one of the fly days. It is not one of the impossible days. It is one of the unbearable ones. Snippets of hope will not save this day. Hugs and comforting words will help, but they will not erase the agony of this ordeal. As it turns out, the only thing bigger than dealing with Carol and Alzheimer's, is dealing with this flawed mental health system. The key is learning to turn the outrage into a positive force for change. We completely understand the safeguards are in place for the protection of the patients. We do not feel that this should be at the cost of desensitizing the staff to the needs of the patients and the needs of those families that are willing to intercede. There must be a middle line. There must be a place for families. There has to be some intermediary to represent both sides.

Saturday, May 22nd

These are some of the things that we feel must be addressed about the process. Some things cannot be changed without dire consequences to the protection of older citizens. Some things can be changed, and should be. I am sure that the process of changing these things will be every bit as educational as this one. I will make sure to save some room in my head for that. Although, there are times I am quite sure there is not any room left. Part of the reason for keeping this journal is so that when this is finally done, we can look back over what happened and see the places where change is needed. The relief of being through the process will try to erase the bad parts. That is just human nature. Our minds want to focus on the good and forget the bad. We need to remember the bad to insure that it does not happen again. I am not sure what will become of these words, but I hope that they might be a help to others that find themselves in the middle of these tall weeds. I hope that we are marking a path.

It is my earnest hope that no one will have go through what we are going through. Human nature as it is though, I am sure someone will. Looking back over this as we go, I can see that there will be much more to educate myself about. There is a variety of avenues that this journey may take. This effort is filled with blind alleys that promise to be your salvation. A map is as much for telling you where not to go, as it is to direct you down the right path. No matter your intentions, you will find yourself against a brick wall somewhere. In that moment, we hope that our experience can help. In the end, when Carol is safe and cared for, this will be the extension of our plight. We will wipe the sweat from our brows and we will sleep a little easier. Well, we will sleep as easy as any parent with kids out in the world will.

Let me share with you my theory on worry. Worry, is when you think about something and you cannot do anything else. The worry controls your every action and thought. This is as deadly as it sounds. Concern, is when you think about something and you still go to work and still cook supper. I guess that is worry-lite.

Most of the time, we are concerned to very concerned about this nightmare. There are times when worry slips in and everything around us stops. It is frightening. It is overwhelming. It is choking at times. Whatever healthy source of comfort you may have, hold to it. You need to be as healthy and as strong as you can possibly be. This is for you as well as those around you that depend on you.

It is yard sale day here. It is almost 80° out there. It does not seem like a good day for having a yard sale or a good day for going to yard sales. Perhaps it is just us. Tired comes a lot faster these days. Stress depletes the body of several essential vitamins. We are taking extra vitamins these days. Who knows if they are helping or not? We are probably soaking up and expending the added effect as fast as we put it in.

Tammy visited Carol today. She was about the same as yesterday. She is still disoriented. She is still scared. She does not understand what is going on. All attempts to assure her are wasted. She tells us not to put ourselves out. She worries that we will incur hurt if we pursue this. I wonder sometimes why she thinks this. Perhaps it is just part of her dementia. Maybe she is just misunderstanding something the doctors tell her. Tammy assures me that it is just how Carol is. She has always worried about authorities.

Sierra is babysitting tonight and taking Kyle with her. That leaves Tammy, Chelsea, and I to fend for ourselves. We took in a Stephen King movie. We had a great time. On our way home, we passed some friends coming out of a restaurant. I gave them a call on the cell phone. They had just finished supper with mutual friends, Brandy and Rob. Brandy lives just down the road from us, so we stopped at their house. It was good to chat. The conversation turned to current events. We gave them the short version. Everyday we add people to the number that are in our small world. Nat and Sid were there. Tomorrow, Nat is moving to Portland, Oregon. We will miss her.

We came home to get a gift for Nat. I had promised her one of my sunset photos previously. It was a good night to make good on that promise. After we dropped it off, we came home. We had a bite to eat. I think it is time to put this day to bed.

Sunday, May 23rd

We kind of slept in. It was eight thirty before I got out of bed. Tammy was an hour or so later. We did not do much this morning. I grilled burgers on the grill outside for lunch. I mowed part of the back yard prior to grilling. While grilling I showed Kyle how to mow. He likes learning bigger chores. It gives him a sense of being more important.

There are so many things going on in which he is completely unable to assist. I know Kyle must get frustrated. He is too young to visit Carol. There is not anything about this in which he can really help. He gets lost in the details sometimes. He is not ignored. He gets his share of attention. He makes sure of that. Still, he knows that he cannot do much about this. When we were on the porch almost two weeks ago and Carol was cussing me, Kyle stood right beside me. He kept hugging me and touching my beard. In his own way, he was protecting me.

It is not as hard for the rest of the kids. They have a greater understanding and they can go and have gone with us to visit Carol. We do not know how it affects them, but feel that it is much healthier to include them. They need to see the conditions and frustrations to better understand how we feel. In this, they share part of this with us.

Evening

Tammy has gone to visit Carol. After visiting, she is going to the grocery. She feels terrible because she does not want to go to Eastern State Mental Hospital. It is a depressing place. I can almost understand how some do not have many visitors. I do not condone leaving a loved one in a place like that, but one must have great determination to go every day. The on call doctor told us that most of the patients do not have anyone. They only get their caring from the staff. From all that I have seen of Gragg 1, they do not get much caring at all. One never comes out of there happy with the visit.

Tammy called me from ESMH. She said there was someone there that wanted to talk to me. I talked to Carol for a while. She wants to keep me, but Tammy ain't going for it. When we finished talking, I got an idea. I went to the front porch where Kyle was sitting and called them back. Kyle talked to Carol. This is the first time she and he have talked since the Monday night that the sheriffs took her away. That was the night he was protecting me. I wanted him to hear her sounding more like Carol. Kyle thinks she sounds better. He thinks things will be better soon.

Next week will bring many changes. School will be out on Wednesday. Our hopes are that we will be bringing Carol home on Tuesday. On June fifth, Ronnie is supposed to be here to pick up the kids. He is taking them to Florida for a month. His summer fun is our summer break. The timing is good. It will give us time to get Carol situated into a new living environment.

There will also be time for us to recharge our batteries. While our 'alone time' has suffered slightly during this, the quality of our time is still as precious as ever. Tammy says she does not know what she would do if I were not here to help her. I married Tammy and all of the extremes of her life. I did not walk into this with my eyes closed. I walked into it with my heart open. It is still open. This has not changed who we are. This has strengthened the bond between us. We collapse at night from exhaustion, but we still collapse together.

When this phase is complete, we will emerge just as strong, if not stronger. This is my faith. I believe in her. She believes in me. We are stronger together than we are separate. Together, we are more than just the sum of our parts.

It is time to fall into bed after one more, long day.

Monday, May 24th

This will be a busy day. There are many phone calls to make and many places to be. Tammy has taken the kids to their respective schools and has gone to physical therapy. I have begun making phone calls.

The first call was to Sherry at Lexington Center For Health & Rehabilitation. I explained to her, who I was, as she had only spoken to Tammy previously. She remembered Tammy and Carol. She said she had tried to call us last week, but did not get an answer. I explained the situation we were in with ESMH and asked if I could get a letter from her stating that they would accept Carol and that she was, in fact, on the waiting list. She explained that another company had just bought LCHR. They have a new name, but she would be glad to write me the letter. I gave her my cell number to call me back later today.

The second call was to Susan at Royal Manor. Susan was not in. I asked if there was someone doing Susan's job while she was not there. They connected me with Margaret, head of nursing. I explained the situation to her and asked if we could get a letter from them about Carol being on their waiting list. Margaret began back peddling faster than a dyslexic dog in a shallow pond. She explained that she only had two male beds available, which we knew. The letter need only state that Carol is on their waiting list. She expressed concern that if Eastern State Mental Hospital wanted to keep her, then there must be a reason. She said that Eastern State was a great facility and was hard to get into. I told her that ESMH was dirty, was reeking of urine, and was not a great place. She suggested I call Susan in the morning. She should be in at 7:45AM.

Tammy is back from PT. She has taken over the phone. She called Judge Turners office about the disposition of Carol's case. They told us to fax the papers showing the emergency guardianship. Those would be presented to the Judge in the morning. We could call back on Friday to find out the ruling on the case.

Tammy then called Eastern State Mental Hospital about having Carol's papers faxed to Homestead Nursing home. They need the social workers note, the doctor's notes, and the floor nurses notes. She then called to talk to the director of ESMH to see if we can override Dr. Hawthorne. Randy Moeler called about mail that Carol received at ESMH. Tammy told him to leave it at G1 and she would pick it up during her daily visit.

Tammy called the Doctor to get Sierra in to see them about her rash. They told her that they did not have any appointments until August.

Melissa Pierce has just returned Tammy's earlier call. She did not seem to think that it would be necessary to fax any papers to Homestead Nursing, since Carol was going to be committed to Eastern State. This was not the right thing to say to Tammy. Tammy assured her that we were going to stop Dr. Hawthorne's efforts to have Carol committed. She told her of Hawthorne's refusal to return our calls. She let her know that we had left messages for Dr. Luctifeld, Director of Eastern State Mental Hospital, as well. It seems he spends a lot of time in meetings.

Tammy asked Melissa what Eastern State's interest was in keeping Carol. It, certainly, is not for her well-being. It is not for the fact that she cannot be cared for elsewhere. It is not for the fact that we cannot care for her. These are not true facts. Tammy assured her that we would be there to stop this. We will not allow Carol to live in filth.

Melissa seems to have done a flip-flop. She now does not think it is necessary to send or release any paperwork. It is premature, she says, because Carol is going to be committed and will not be going to a nursing home.

I called David Kaplan, a friend and lawyer. He said they had the cart before the horse. We can ask for a continuance because of their reluctance to assist us in our efforts to get Carol placement.

Tammy called and finally reached Dr. Hawthorne. When asked why he felt Carol needed to be committed, he told her about the placement issue. She told him that we had nursing homes lined up to take Carol. When she told him that she was a mental health tech, he said, "I don't care what you are", and hung up the phone. This is quite the professional bunch. NOT.

I, then, called ESMH to speak to the Director. I told his secretary, Joyce, to have him call me and explain why he professional staff hangs up when asked a question. I asked her to have him explain to me why his wards are filthy and reeking of urine. I told her that he could contact my attorney or me.

I contacted Sen. McConnell's office. They put me on the trail of the Cabinet for Health & Human Services. There, I spoke to Dana Abbott. She was shocked by the situation as I explained it. She then, in turn, gave me the numbers for Kentucky Guardianship Services and for the Office of the Inspector General.

The KGS was only able to offer advice. The person I spoke to there (I did not catch her name) told me to keep a paper trail. She told me to make sure that I informed the judge of everything we have been told by Dr. Hawthorne and ESMH.

The second call reaped more benefits. While I was on the phone with them, Dan Luctifeld returned my call. Tammy is on the phone with him while I talk to the Inspector General's office. The office I called was in Louisville. They gave me the number of the Lexington office and told me to ask for Connie Payne. Connie was aghast about the report I gave her. She is assigning an investigator to check it. While this does very little to help with our immediate situation, it does give one a sense of accomplishing something against the brick wall of indifference. Everyone I have talked to has wished me the best of luck.

Tammy's call with Luctifeld was not as pleasant. He told her the Hawthorne felt that it would be unsafe for Carol to be with us. I fail to see how he would know this, since he had never spoken to us until this morning. Luctifeld said that he understood the Hawthorne had been in contact with us all along. Tammy explained that he understood wrong. He refused to overturn Hawthorne's decision. He said that best he could do would be to have another psychiatrist examine her. When asked about the deplorable conditions on the floor, his response was, "We have housekeeping."

Interestingly enough, we found out this morning that the court date had been changed to Thursday. No one from the hospital bothered to inform us. We also found out this morning that Carol had a new court appointed attorney. His name is Ben Cabway. I called Mr. Cabway and explained to him that situation. He, too, is shocked. He says he will ask for a jury trial, if necessary. We have a meeting with him tomorrow at 3:30 PM. He wants to make sure we are there for the hearing. He also wants all the information we have gathered concerning this case.

There is still a call to be made to David Gottfried. Hang on, while I call. Ok, David was surprised at the turn of events. He did suggest that we sign a 'hippa' letter to have her records released. Then ESMH has no course except to comply.

AMAZING! While on the phone with David Gottfried, Melissa Pierce with Eastern State Mental Hospital called Tammy's phone to tell us that we can take Carol home today at 6PM. If Eastern State thinks that this is the end of our involvement in their affairs, they are sadly mistaken. We have only begun our crusade. Getting Carol out of there was only our first priority. Once that is accomplished, we can concentrate on the rest of our complaints and observations.

I do not know why they suddenly changed their mind, nor do I care. I do wonder if it was the profundity of our efforts, or the number of our calls, to them and others. We will concentrate out efforts more on getting Carol placed, but we will not forget what we have come through to get here. There is still a 'recompense of reward.'

I called Ben Cabway to inform him of the hospital's new decision. He was out of the office.

Rachel Hockensmith of The Department of Protection and Advocacy returned Tammy's call of this morning. Tammy apprised them of the situation. They told her that we needed to call the Inspector General's office. She told them we had. They told her that we should call a Senator's office. She told her that I had. They said we were on the right road. Rachel told us to 'shut them down.' They have been trying for years. She asked if we would be willing and available for their efforts to do this. We readily agreed.

I called Wayne Cook to check on the disposition of the petition of the commitment. He told me that it has been discharged. There was no hearing. There is no petition. He did tell me to make sure to give them the name of the doctor of wherever we got Carol placed. This is necessary for the full guardianship petition. That hearing is in July.

ESMH sent home a prescription of Aricept for Carol. We called RiteAid Pharmacy to check on the price. Fifteen pills cost eighty-six dollars and ninety-nine cents. I asked about the Medicare Prescription Discount. The person I was talking to, who kept going somewhere to re-ask my questions, told me that it was not covered. This is odd, seeing as how it is a drug for Alzheimer's. We called Community Action Council to find out any place that helps with prescriptions. They recommended Faith Pharmacy. We left a message for them.

We called Walgreen's Pharmacy. They have the same medicine for seventy-five dollars and ninety-nine cents. The pills are to be taken once a day at bedtime. The pharmacist at Walgreen told us to check at Sam's club. It is seventy-two dollars and seventy-cents.

Tammy is reading over the papers that ESMH send home with Carol. This includes the doctor notes and such. There is one entry on May 22nd, where Carol told the nurse to 'give her a broom or a shovel to clean this place up.' The hospital inadvertently sent home a list of other patients in Carol's papers. These are the things that make you go hmmmm. The doctor that we spoke to on Friday did enter into the record that we were requesting to take Carol home with us. She noted our concern and caring. She also noted the support from both of us.

The validity of the following is questionable, but deserves a mention. Carol told us there was a sharp dressed man that paid a visit to G1. He could not get in the door because there was a puddle of urine in the doorway. This was after our calls to the Director about the conditions of that ward.

Another day and another lesson learned. We continue to be educated.

Tuesday, May 25th

The first call today is to Faith Pharmacy about getting Carol help with her prescription. They only fill prescriptions on Saturday. We will need a referral from a social worker. They have a part time social worker there. Tammy made appointment for 1PM today. On Saturday, we have to be at the corner of Elm Tree and Seventh Street to get the prescription. They start filling them at 9AM. The woman told us to be there early. Sometimes, there is a line.

The second call was to Ben Cabway at Legal Aid. It is eight thirty AM. He has not made it to the office yet. I left him a message to call me. I am sure that he is aware that the hearing has been dropped, but I want to thank him for his fervor. I also want to find out the results of his visit with Hawthorne.

Yesterday I talked with a friend that previously worked for the Herald Leader. I asked about contacts that she might still have that could help get this story told. She says, she has been gone too long and most to all of her contacts has moved on to other places. She suggested calling one of the local TV news stations. Later that evening, we spoke again in a three-way conversation with a friend of hers that is an acquaintance of mine. Michael works with a print company that does a lot of advertising with the Herald. He might have a source. He will be checking this morning and getting back to me on it.

While taking care of Carol is our number one priority, the outrage of the way we were treated is fresh. I cannot remember where the line came from originally, but I keep hearing it in my head. "We will not go quiet into the dark night."

It is about twenty minutes until ten o'clock. We are about to embark on a journey. I remember when I was twenty and married. Kaye and I would decide to go somewhere, such as, the store, or Florida. We would take five minutes to gather whatever we needed for that trip and toss it in the car and go. Then Audrey came along. Things changed greatly. There were no more spur of the moment trips to Florida. Even trips to the store changed. There was so much more to consider now. There were bottles to prepare and pack. There were diapers to pack. There were the wipes, and the powder, and the juice, and all the other things that babies need. This made every trip an adventure.

This is somewhat similar. Carol requires her own preparation. We have to consider whether we can take her with us to where ever we are going. If not, one of us has to go and one of us has to stay. We have to plan for more time. Carol moves slower than we do. We have to figure what we are doing and where we are going to make the best of the trip out. We cannot just take ourselves out to the truck and go. Oh yeah, factor into all of this that we are babysitting Ian today as well. We have age considerations on both sides of the age spectrum.

We will try to take copies to homestead and pick up a now not needed letter from one nursing home. We have to stop by ARC. We will stop by my parent's house. I have to return the camera and take him the lease from the apt upstairs. We need to return movies we rented on Sunday. Then we will make a Wal-Mart trip. Sierra wants to order a cake for Jordan's birthday. Sounds like a fun trip. Wanna come?

We are back. That was a fun trip. Carol met my parents. She loved my mom. We then went to one of the nursing homes that wrote us a letter stating that Carol was on their waiting list. When we pulled in, I noticed there were no signs pointing out that it were a nursing home. Still, Carol knew what it was. She got defensive immediately. We pointed out that we were not dropping her off.

From there we went to ARC to pick up job description for Tammy. We may or may not need these things, but we do not want to ignore the efforts. We want to acknowledge that we needed their help and that we are grateful for every scrap of assistance. Carol was confused about our trips. She still insisted that she needed to go to the house and get some money from Jim. Tammy reminded her that Jim is in Florida and that she is in Kentucky. She remembers sometimes.

While Tammy was inside the office, Carol talked to me. She was agitated that I did not tell her earlier that she was in Kentucky. I stated that I had told her numerous times. I told her that no matter how many times we tell her, she is going to forget. She went one to tell me that 'this' is not going to work. 'This' is whatever she is trying to reason in her head and cant recall. 'This' is that elusive thought that she can't grasp. She uses the word all the time. When you try to pin her down on exactly what 'this' is, she tells you, "You know what this is." She is not stupid. She is struggling with this sickness. 'This' is everything that is outside of her grasp.

Carol, again, reiterated that she wanted her own place. She wanted her stuff. This is a daily thing. Sometimes, it is an hourly thing. This is where it seems exasperating. I told her very plainly that she was going to do it our way. I explained to her that her choices were simple. She can do it our way or she can go back to the place from which we rescued her. At that moment, she did not remember Eastern State Mental Hospital.

She worries about my driving. We were on our way to my parents. The posted speed limit was thirty-five MPH. I was doing close to forty. She estimated my speed at sixty. She told Tammy that she was going to get out because she was worried. I decided that I would fix the child lock on her door so that it could only be opened from outside.

Tammy says that it is like having an overly intelligent two year old. The thoughts are there. The rationality to put them together has gone somewhere else. While I am writing this, Carol is trying to do the dishes. I told her that we would take care of the dishes. She insists on doing them. I told her that she needed to wait, since not everyone has had supper yet. Sierra has not eaten. She said that she would just stack them. Then she proceeded to try to wash them. She said everyone has had supper. It was almost one minute since I told her Sierra had not eaten. She is washing them now. I am wondering if she is rinsing them this time. Last time she tried, she washed then and put them in the drainer from the soapy water. Need a maid?

We have heard others call it 'old timers'. I think it is 'young timers'. She acts like Kyle. He is eight years old and very intelligent. As smart as he is, though, it occasionally works against him. He thinks he is able to do more than he is actually capable of doing. He will tear up something trying to use it, because he really does not know how. I have to give him detailed directions for using the computer when we are not around.

He tries to understand subjects beyond his reach. It is fun to listen to him expound his theories about the end of the dinosaurs, or aliens, or religion. Having Kyle around has trained us for Carol.

At some point during the day, the Office of the Inspector General called. We were out and got the message too late to return the call. I will call them in the morning.

Wednesday, May 26th

Tammy took the kids to school today for the final time of this session. She took Sierra with her to allow her to see Jordan. She took Carol as well. They went with her to PT. Sierra babysat.

While they were gone, I made necessary calls to my health insurance provider. Kaye called me yesterday about Heather's upcoming medical tests. They will be covered. I also called my prescription coverage to check on the deductible. Mine has been met. Heather's has not been met.

After I got all of those calls out of the way, I returned Rita Satterly's call. She is with the Office of the Inspector General. Rita told me that she visited Eastern State Mental Hospital and spoke with them about our concerns. She addressed the medical part of the complaint first. Eastern State's explanation was that Hawthorne was concerned for Carol's safety. When she transferred to another ward, a new doctor, Corales, decided it was safe for her to go home. It was interesting that when we tried to get her released from the new ward, we were told that Dr. Hawthorne had to OK it. Suddenly, it is out of Hawthorne's hands and a new doctor is making those decisions.

Rita then addressed the issue of the wards sanitary conditions. She saw none of the things we spoke of on the phone. She did say that housekeeping was there cleaning when she visited. Of course, they were. They knew that we had complained. I told her of the interchange that Tammy overheard between an employee and a patient. The employee was telling a patient, "You missed the time to eat. Now you won't eat until tomorrow." She said that would not be acceptable. She asked if we wanted to file a complaint about that statement. I told her that it would not do any good.

Abuse and neglect almost have to be witnessed by the official to be considered. It is our word against theirs. When we expressed that to Dan Luctifeld, his response was one of disbelief. When administrators refuse to acknowledge the possibility that such neglect and abuse are possible, there is little hope for change.

I thanked Rita for returning my call and letting me know the results. She assured me there were several agencies that were watching places like Eastern State Mental Hospital very closely. I do hope that ours is an isolated incident. Somehow, my head and heart are not convinced.

Tammy got her TENS unit today. UPS delivered it. I read up on it and attached it to her wrist. A little adjusting and she is pain free. Maybe this will allow her more usage of that wrist and therefore loosen it up a bit. The pain is, as always, an inhibitor.

Carol has been cleaning in the kitchen to feel useful. She did the dishes. The silverware was in the drainer, unwashed. One spoon still had mayonnaise on it. The plates were still dirty, but in the drainer also. She put a pot that she had washed in the deep fryer. The deep fryer was full of oil. She swept up the floor and left the dirt in piles. Then, she used a knife to scrape the floors. She rearranged the refrigerator. Tammy had trouble finding the things she wanted.

She explained to Carol that she needed to leave things in the kitchen alone. She did not need to move things from one place to another. As Tammy puts it, two women in one kitchen do not work. I can understand that as I am in the kitchen all the time as well. I love to cook and hate when I open the cabinet to get a spice or can and it is not where I put it. I hate having to search every cabinet for the wok. It is frustrating.

The mail carrier came while Carol was on the porch and gave Tammy mail. He said, "Carol Young?" asking if her mail was to come here. Tammy took the mail and opened a hospital bill for Carol. Carol was upset that Tammy opened her mail. She had to explain that we were taking care of these things now.

Then there was the "N" word. The young man that just rented the apt upstairs is mixed. He has been going back and forth moving things in and getting the utilities set. Carol wanted to know whom that 'nigger boy' was that kept coming over. Tammy told her that word was not acceptable in our house. She said she could not help it. That was the way she was raised. Tammy then told her that she could help it. She asked her if she planned to be ignorant all of her life. It is quite the adjustment having Carol here.

Carol went to sit on the porch. She gets antsy in the house after long periods. She wanted to know if she could take the broom outside and sweep the porch. Tammy allowed that. Anything to keep her occupied and feeling useful is a good thing, within reason. She stays on the porch. She is afraid of the traffic here. She came in shortly ago. It is storming outside. The thunder and lightning bother her. Tammy is napping on the couch and Carol is sitting quietly in the chair, dozing. I am online while writing this. Every now and then, the computer says, "You've got mail." Carol says that is nice to know.

She just told me that she was just sitting quietly. She has not hatched anything, just sitting, she says. Carol is rather funny when she is not confused. There are glimpses of Carol every now and then. Somewhere beneath the years of anger and the ravages of this disease, is a smart and kind woman. This 'Carol' is the only one I have ever known. I guess that is why it does not bother me as much as it bothers Tammy. It does hurt me to see her suffer so much with trying to reconcile random thoughts. Tammy, on the other hand, knew her when she was sharp. She saw her when she worked and carried responsibility. Tammy is angry with the Alzheimer's disease. She is angry with Carol as well. She hates that she let Jim Young break her down. She blames this as much as the disease. He broke her strength, and she kept coming back to him.

I guess if this disease has one redeeming quality, it is that the patient does not know how bad they are. Carol does not realize how sick she is. She does not know that her mind is not firing right. She does not realize that she does not know what she does not know. It is a terrible thing to find a bright spot in this inhumane condition. If there is one, that is it. That bright spot still does not compare to the darkness of the sickness.

Thursday, May 27th

Carol has begun the "I have got to go home" thing again. I guess the most frustrating part of this is explaining. It gets exasperating at times explaining subjects to your children, but you have hope. They will learn. This is not the case with Carol. She is not going to learn. She is not going to remember eventually.

Today, she also thought that Mary, her mother, was in Lexington and she needed to go there. I explained that she was in Lexington. She told me she was not talking about this Lexington. She was talking about the Lexington where Momma was. She told me that I did not know about Lexington. She knew all about it because she was born and raised there. She was delighted when I told her that I was born in Lexington, as well.

She wanted a paper and pencil to write down some things she needed to remember. She wrote about a court date that she thinks she has. She talks about 'that man' that ruined it all. This is not Jim Young. She had an accident in which she damaged a man's truck. He sued and wanted her to make payments to him. She did not have insurance at the time. She received a ticket for driving with a revoked license. She was also charged with financial responsibility. This means there was a lawsuit filed for the damages. Carol talks about this man coming to the house and asking her for one hundred fifty dollars a week. According to her, this was the beginning of all her troubles.

It is funny that Carol tries to play me when Tammy tells her one thing. She tries to get me to agree to something else. It never works, but she cannot remember exactly what Tammy said. Therefore, she thinks she has done something. In all actuality, I have agreed with what Tammy said to begin with.

Carol wants to make sure the nursing home she goes into has doors that she can walk out. She still does not understand that she is not going to be able to just walk out and go to town. She cannot grasp the idea that she is not going to be working as she was in Florida. She tells us repeatedly that she is going to get a job. Today, she found the classified section of a newspaper. She is holding on to it. She might be able to find a job that she can do. It does us no good to explain to her that she cannot work. She just does not understand that she cannot work. She does not understand that no one would hire her.

On the brighter side, she is sleeping better and more. That is probably because of the reduction of stress. This house, with all of its chaos, is still less stressful than the house she shared with Jim in Florida and much less so than Eastern State Mental Hospital.

This afternoon, she asked Tammy why we brought her up here in the first place.

Friday, May 28th

I woke up early this morning. We were up late because of the storms. There were tornados that touched down in Lexington. The weather was the news. I went to bed around one AM, but was up a couple hours later as the second wave went through. I did not hear of any more touchdowns. Then I woke up an hour or so before Tammy needed to get out of bed.

I woke her up in time to get ready for physical therapy. We kept it quiet so that we would not awaken Carol. This way Tammy could go to therapy alone. Carol woke up and asked about Tammy. I told her she had gone to see the doctor.

While she was waiting for Tammy and the headache powders, we chatted. She talked about Jim dropping her off and leaving us to provide her care. This was amazing. Mostly, she does not recollect those events at all.

We are still in waiting mode. We are still going behind Carol and taking the dishes out of the drainer, which she has washed. She was in the kitchen knocking around. I asked Kyle to check on her when he got me a bottle of water. She was preparing a cup of coffee. She got agitated at Kyle for asking what she was doing. She got a little sarcastic with him. Kyle did not take it very well. He complained about having her here all the time.

This is one of my worries. I do not want the kids to resent Carol for the changes we have been required to make. Generally, there needs to be someone with or near her about ninety percent of the time. Tammy and I cannot always be on the porch, or at home. The kids have been picking up the slack. While we appreciate everything they do, we do not want them to be angry with Carol. The girls, for the most part, just ignore her comments or her zaniness.

Tammy and I went to the movies this afternoon. It was a solo trip. It was our need to be away from the house and everyone in it. It was a nice break. Before going, we told Carol that we were going out for a while. She asked if she could ride along. Tammy told her that she could not go with us this time. We were about to leave the house when I noticed Carol crying. I asked if she was ok. (She has mood swings.) She told me that she was, in fact, not Ok. She knew, she said, where we were going. We were "going to go there and do that thing that we need to get done so we can put her into a nursing home". I assured her that we were not going to any nursing homes. "We are going to the movies," I said. "No, you are not going to the movies. It is in the day." I found out later from Tammy that Carol thinks movies are only shown at night. Again, I assured her that we were indeed going to the movies and they we would be back in a couple hours.

Of course, a trip to the movies would not be complete with a few phone calls from the kids. I ignored the first two from Sierra's cell phone. When the number showed up as the house phone, however, I answered. It was no emergency. It was Kyle. He did not know we were where we were. I solved his dilemma and we were back to alone.

Sierra left a message. She needed cigs. Just as the movie ended, she called again. Now, she needs cigs and socks. We stopped at the house, got her socks, and stopped by the drug store to get her cigs. Carol did ride along with us. We then grabbed a couple movies at blockbuster and did a little grocery shopping at Kroger for me to cook supper tonight.

Before supper, I explained to Carol the chore thing. Where she was, she had to do it all and there was always some chore do. Here, with five people doing the chores, there was much more 'free' time. If she does the dishes, that leaves the person responsible for them with nothing to do. She did seem to understand this, for the moment, and asked to be placed on the rotation.

Why do I add these details? It is to help myself remember and to help you to understand in some small way what goes on in this world of Alzheimer's. Just as they say that alcoholics are not the only victims of their drinking, neither is the patient the only one affected. Unless you have been canonized as the patron saint of patience, you will become exasperated. Do not beat yourself up over it. Carol thinks that everything said, is being said to her. She responds to everything said. She talks. She talks a lot. Perhaps, it is her mind spilling. Perhaps, she just says whatever comes to mind. Regardless, she talks a lot. Did I mention that she talks a lot?

Saturday, May 29th

It is Saturday afternoon and for the tenth time today, we have explained to Carol that she is going to live in Kentucky. She cannot reconcile it in her mind that she will not be living in Florida and Kentucky at the same time. She rehashes the same worries and concerns about every hour. She wants to call people in Florida to take her there. She does not understand that she will not be living in Florida. She talks about different ones that will come get her. We explained to her that we were looking for a place here. We even mentioned the several nursing homes that we have contacted. One of those has an address on Versailles Rd. When we tell her that she is going to be here in KY, she rants that we need to make up our minds, because we just told her she might be on Versailles Rd.

It is very selective as to the new information that she retains. Generally, she eventually forgets it all. There are moments that she remembers pieces. They do not make sense to her. She gets irritated. She lashes out verbally. She is offended that we keep track of her whereabouts. If anyone asks where she is going, she reacts angrily. I do not worry when she is short with me, but I do worry about Kyle. Tammy says that if she were angry enough, she would smack him. I will have to caution him about asking her where she is going. He will need to just watch her or find one of us. The girls can pretty much fend for themselves.

She keeps telling us that she is "not going to be treated like a GD dog". This seems to be one of her favorite sayings. Tammy says that she was mean before Alzheimer's and it has not done much to improve this. Tammy tells me stories about her childhood that proves that point. There is a term for what Carol has. It goes beyond Alzheimer's disease. She is emotionally retarded. Her emotions stopped developing when she was younger. Even though she worked and operated her own business, she stayed at a child's level emotionally. She has a dependency on Jim Young because of it.

Here we go on round one hundred thirty-seven. One more time we explain as she runs from one point to another. Carol jumps from Jim, to her furniture, to her mother, to finding her a house, to not wanting to be in a nursing home, and so forth. Obsessive-compulsive behavior seems to run in the family. The biggest problem is, with her scattered thoughts, she will obsess for five seconds on one subject and then move on. It is impossible to make any headway like that. As soon as you get close to making a point, she switches channels.

To explain to her just how bad she is; I asked her my name. She did not know what it was. About an hour ago while we were waiting for Tammy to return to the truck, I showed her my old license. She commented on my name. She told me that she did not realize that my last name was Simpson. "Well, it is now that you have married Tammy", she told me. She does not know what her daughter's last name was. Now, just over one hour later, she does not know my name. She knows who I am, as far as Tammy's husband, but that is all.

Sunday, May 30th

She was up and dressed when I came out of the bedroom around 8:30 AM. Kyle was up as well. Carol fixed a cup of coffee and went to the front porch. She came in later to tell me she had been talking to a new friend. She 'lives on Versailles Rd'. In the course of the conversation, she told me about her living across town and her house being right up the road. These inconsistencies are warning signs. She does not even recognize that statements she makes are contradictory.

Kyle pulled the center cushion off the couch while playing. Carol noticed that there were some things under it and decided she just had to clean that. While scrapping it all together, she was talking to Kyle. He told me that he "could not take it one more day." He does have a tendency to over dramatize. I explained to him, privately, that all he has to do is ignore her when she is like that. I further explained that Carol is obsessive-compulsive, as is Tammy, as is he. All people tend to obsess about various things. Carol is unable to recognize this in herself and therefore allows these obsessions to rule her life.

Obsession, in and of itself, is not the problem. Her meanness is not so much a problem on its own either. The coupling of these factors with Alzheimer's creates the problem.

Evening

Calvert, Carol's son called this evening. She began trying to convince him to allow her to come live with him. She sprayed her scattered facts to no avail. I felt sorry for him.

He and I spoke for a bit before the phone went to Carol. We talked about the need to find time away from the situation. He told me that he and Karin, his wife, took their dog for many walks. Everyone got healthier. He does not want Carol in Arizona.

Monday, May 31st Memorial Day

The day was quiet in the morning, other than Carol's usual talking. The storms of the last couple of days seem to have faded. The thunderstorms and tornados have done their damage and moved on. Last night around one AM, I checked the basement. There was about eight inches of water standing. This morning that has increased to twelve inches. Not much more and the water heaters burners will be underwater. After making a few calls and discovering that everyone in Lexington either needs or has just purchased a sump pump, we are off to buy a sump pump. Carol and Kyle are our tag-a-longs. After purchasing a pump, we drive to Dad's house to pick up a reimbursement check.

Tammy and I hung out in the back yard while the pump did its job. It was nice. It was away from the traffic and mostly alone. It was good to talk about sump pumps and wet basements without having to repeat or explain everything. This has put a strain on our conversations. Tammy and I talk about anything and everything and love doing so. When Carol is around, that is difficult to do. She has to comment on everything said. She imagines that every word is directed toward her. Tammy says at times, she just wishes that Carol would stop talking.

Later in the afternoon, the kids asked if they could go for a walk around the block. It was clearly stated that it was going to be a walk 'around the block'. Carol asked if she could go with them. It seemed harmless enough. We gave Chella the cell phone in case something happened. They made it to the corner. Chella calls. Carol does not want to walk around the block. She wants to come back to the house. Her legs hurt and she cannot walk that far. Tammy drives to pick them up. They had walked about a block.

When Carol got into the car, she made a comment about 'that bitch over there' and motioned toward Chelsea. This was not the right thing to say. On the 'long' ride home, Carol told Tammy that she was tired of "being treated like a damn dog". They were still fussing when they came in the door. Tammy told me what had happened. She had to get away from Carol. She was going to the porch or Carol was. With Tammy out of the room, I confronted Carol about her actions. She did not remember saying it. It was about five minutes after it happened.

I told her, that kind of behavior was not going to be tolerated. She began to stammer, stutter, and deny ever saying anything like it. She claims that she has never claimed that we treat her like a dog. She has, many times. She tried to tell me that she had a sickness. This is after denying for weeks that she has any sickness. When all other arguments failed, she reverted to blaming everything on Jim Young.

I have noticed this in her. Carol does not take the blame for anything. When it is convenient to blame her condition, she has it. When it is easier to blame Jim Young, she blames him. None of this is her fault. Nothing that has happened in her life is her fault. This is not a condition of the Alzheimer's. This is a product of her emotional retardation.

Chelsea noticed how upset Tammy was and asked if there was anyway I could take her out this evening. We did have to go to Nicholasville, so we took a solo trip. Carol stayed with the kids. It was good to drive alone for thirty minutes. The visit with Audrey was good as well. We loved seeing the grandkids. Another thirty-minute drive home was heaven. The kids and Carol were still on the porch when we arrived home.

Carol came in and started going through her purse. This is a regular thing. She is constantly taking papers out, looking at them, and putting them back. It is ok when she does this. I noticed that she is quiet except for mumbling to herself while doing it. She finished her purse excavation and went to the kitchen for a glass of water.

When she returned, she informed me that she needed to find a way to go tomorrow and fill her prescription. She found it <u>finally</u> while digging in her purse. I asked what drug it was for. "Xanax," she replied. I asked what it was for. She replied, "For me and nobody else". I clarified my question. She decided that I needed to see the prescription for myself because I just did not understand. She is back in the dark caverns of her purse, searching. She does have a prescription for Xanax in her purse. It is dated, 2003. When questioned about it, it was Jim Young's fault.

She lacks the capability to reason logically. She insisted that she had seen Dr. Idiculla just a month ago. I told her that we had talked to him. He said she had not been in the office since November 2002. She said that was a 'goddam' lie. Therefore, I asked her if Dr. Idiculla was lying. She said he was not. I said, "So, you haven't been there in a year and a half". She insisted still that she was there last month. In her head, this makes sense: Dr. Idiculla is telling the truth when he says she has not been there in a year and a half, even though that is a lie.

She continued to go on about it. Then she switched to momma, then to furniture, then to that lying sonovabitch Jim. I told her to hush. She would try to talk and I would immediately tell her to hush. She would still try. Finally, I told her she could talk all she wanted but no one was going to listen any more. She muttered on a little bit but got no response. She eventually hushed. I went to the porch and informed Tammy and the kids that they were not to acknowledge her talking. It works. Of course, I lost my chance at sainthood, but the peace is worth it. Tomorrow, she will not remember any of it.

Tuesday, June 1st

I woke up at seven AM to Carol yelling to tell us the phone was ringing. I came into the living room. It was not the phone ringing; it was Tammy's cell phone alarm going off. Carol drifted back off to sleep. I stayed up. Kyle got up around eight-thirty AM. The doorbell rang at around nine. It was Heather. She was between tests. I woke Chelsea and Sierra, briefly. It is now 9:20, and Tammy, Carol, Kyle, and I are up. Carol is quiet. Tammy says she can hear the ticking. We will see what the day brings.

Tammy has calls to make at 10. She is getting a social worker for Carol. At 1PM, she has an appointment to apply for Medicaid. She says that I will have to push her to do the nursing home necessities.

On a side note, the kids are all out of school. Kyle brought home all his clothes that he had left at school on May 26th. He has been enjoying his summer vacation and playing a lot with the new kid in the apt upstairs. While he was playing upstairs this morning, my doorbell chimed. I answered the door to a woman in her late twenties. She asked for Kyle Morgan. I asked her if she knew the Kyle was only eight years old. I figured they had picked up his name off some list and did not realize that he was a kid. She assured me that she knew that. I asked what her business was with Kyle as I was his dad. She was looking for me.

She wanted to know why Kyle had not been to school. I told her we thought school was out. She informed me that Johnson, on the alternative calendar, did not get out of school until June 8th. I guaranteed her that Kyle would be at school in the morning.

When Kyle came downstairs for his check in, I asked him about this. Knowing that he was caught, he confessed that he let us believe school was out because he did not want to go back. I told him to go back upstairs to play. When Tammy returned we would talk about his punishment. He had that 'I'm sunk' look on his face. I called Tammy to let her know what was happening. We got the laughing part out of the way then. You cannot seriously scold your child while you are laughing at the audacity of their offence.

Tammy has returned from the Medicaid office. It appears that the person lost the appointment. They waited for hours to sit in the office with Ms Roach. She conducted the appointment from the pissed position. She seemed to be aggravated that she had to do her job. Even if she forgot the appointment, she still had to be in the office. Everyone was there, so why not just do the job the Government pays you to do.

My work is seasonal at times. During my off times, I would collect unemployment. Most of the kind people at the unemployment office were as helpful as they could be. Every now and then, however, I would run into one of those civil servants that had the attitude that they were writing that check out of their own account. It never understood that then. I cannot understand it now. The contractor for whom I was working pays unemployment. The Government pays for Medicaid. Approving or denying any one individual is not going to increase or lessen the tax burden of that government worker.

It seems that some of these workers do not know their own rules. Ms. Roach told Tammy that she might not qualify because of our income. Tammy told her that Carol was allowed to stay somewhere for thirty days without being considered a resident. There is a catch 22 here. Apparently, according to Ms. Roach, she cannot get Medicaid until she gets into a nursing home but cannot get into a nursing home until she gets Medicaid. This is not true. Many elderly people not in nursing home qualify for Medicaid. It makes you wonder how many are out there deserving of it but denied by this type of ignorance. When it is all said and done, they input the given information into a computer and that computer determines eligibility based on preset criterion. Just take the information, input it, and go on to the next victim.

Oh yeah, Kyle is grounded at least until the weekend.

Carol asked me if Calvert was going to call back. I told her I did not know that he was supposed to call back. She launched into a 'me and Calvert have things to discuss about me and mamma' discussion. She told me that it was not any of my business. I assured her that if it concerned her placement and her mothers move, it did concern me, since Tammy and I were the ones doing that. She became argumentative about it. I told her we were not discussing this any more. She muttered on about it for about five minutes more with no response from me. It died.

Evening
We finally got Carol to take a shower. She has not taken one since she got here. I do not know if she showered at ESMH. Tammy says they did. It was a daily thing. We tried to get her to take one a few days ago. She was in the bathroom for a bit. The water ran for about a minute. She came out drying her hands. I think that was all she washed. Tammy helped her into the tub. She showed Carol where all the soaps and shampoos were. When Tammy walked out, I heard Carol talking to herself about not needing to wash her hair. I ratted her out. Tammy went in to tell her that she needed to wash her hair. She said. "OK." When she was finished, she came out with dry hair.

One of the reports of Carol's first evaluation stated that she was malodorous. Tammy had to clean the bathroom after Carol's shower because of the odor. While Tammy says that she has never been a bath a day person, she has never been this bad. Tammy has an obsessive-compulsive thing about daily showers for herself. She thinks this may be part of the reason.

The now fresher Carol is asleep on the couch. Another long day has passed into yesterday. My bed is calling my name. I think I will answer.

Wednesday, June 2nd

Kyle is in school. Tammy is running. She finished PT and came home. She left her envelope filled with the papers necessary for the next appt. She ran through like a whirlwind. Carol asked if she could go with her. Tammy rushed her out the door. A quick kiss or two and she was gone.

The Social Security Office was quick. Tammy arrived, let the receptionist know she was there, and sat down. About three minutes later, she was called back for her appointment. Ms. Howard was very pleasant. She worked with Tammy to speed up the process. Tammy was amazed.

When she got home, Tammy laid down for a bit. This week has been long on all of us. Chelsea was asleep on the floor. Carol was asleep on the couch. I woke Tammy up at two-forty. She needed to leave at two-fifty to gather Kyle from school. After getting Kyle, she was going to Leonard's place to pick up her new pet, a Pomeranian named Donavon.

While she was gone, Carol asked me if she could go to Martha's house to visit. Martha lives a couple doors down. I told her that was ok. Then, I asked Chelsea to walk her down there to make sure she made it. A few minutes later, Chelsea comes in telling me that Carol is walking door to door, knocking on doors, looking for her friend. She left Jordan, the 13 year old from upstairs, with her. I told her to go back and I would be out as soon as put on my shoes. In the two minutes it took me to get my shoes on and get out the door, they had disappeared.

I walked to where I thought Martha told me she lived. Jordan was running across the yard. He led me to the back where Carol was arguing with Chelsea. Martha was upset about this. I told Carol that Chelsea was doing as I had asked of her. Martha wanted to know why we had such a tight hold on Carol. I told her it was because she had Alzheimer's and would not remember how to get back to the house. Several of the times we have been out, Carol has not recognized the house when we returned. Martha said she would make sure that Carol made it home.

I told Carol to calm down and I would be back later to bring her home. She assured me that she did not need help getting home. I smiled and left, knowing I would be back in thirty minutes to collect her. About fifteen minutes later Carol came home. She asked if I had five minutes to talk. I told her I did. She proceeded to tell me how embarrassed she was by the actions of those that were there. She did not see why anyone had to be there with her. I told her that I sent Chelsea with her to make sure she was fine, as she complained about her legs hurting yesterday. She could not connect that with why Chelsea was there today. I explained, in vain, that the only person embarrassing anyone was she. If she had any reason to be humiliated, it would be because of her actions.

This became pointless and I abandoned trying to explain it to her. She cannot think in a straight line. She talked for the next fifteen minutes. She did not keep any line of reason for more than three lines. She told me she did not want to stay at the nursing home that she visited yesterday. She was talking about the Medicaid office. She was worried about the long dark hallway. I assured her that we had not taken her to any nursing home for a visit as of yet. Then we digressed into the Jim Young, momma, furniture discussion. Well, we did not. She did.

In the middle of all of this, during the day, I managed to make some Cajun Cole slaw and prepared steaks for grilling out tonight.

Tammy returned with Donavon, Sierra, Kyle, and Jordan. I shared my time with Carol with her. She bathed the dog. When she was finished, we took the grill out and I lost myself in cooking. Sierra put Carol's obsession with cleaning to use. She asked her to help clean her room. Carol was in heaven, until she tried cleaning some of Kyle's things and he objected. Carol was alone in the room. Sierra was on the porch with Jordan. Supper put a temporary stop to the cleaning and, subsequently, to the squabbling.

Carol loved supper, but complained that we fattening her up. She also obsesses about her weight. She ain't big as nothing. She is a size four. Supper finished, cleaning resumed. Tammy corralled all the kids to assist this time.

We are still waiting for word from nursing homes. Carol will have her check tomorrow and we will have something to work with in getting her placed. I hope that we will have word on Medicaid soon. We still need to find a social worker for Carol. The Center for Woman and Children is supposed to call us back on that. The sense of urgency is one thing you cannot share. Everyone has his or her own timetable. Eventually, everything will coincide. Carol will have her place. Mary will be here. The planets will align. Peace will rule the planet. OK, OK, maybe not, but it is a nice thought. I will just settle for some time alone with my wife and explaining things only once.

Thursday, June 3rd

Tammy has PT today and took Carol and Chelsea. Carol got upset while Tammy was at therapy. Leslie, one of the therapists, came back to tell Tammy. When she got out to the waiting area, Carol was cussing someone. Tammy told her to lower her voice. Carol told her that these people did not care. Tammy said that she cared. She got Carol quiet and finished the exercise. She left early because of Carol.

Afterwards, Tammy dropped off my truck payment. Then she went to Homestead Nursing Home to give them copies of Carol's files. They are coming tomorrow to meet the family. They feel it puts everyone in a more comfortable setting to do this in the home.

The mail carrier brought mail for Carol. There was a letter stating that her Medicare was no longer going to be taken out of her Social Security check. This is going to give her a few dollars more per month. Martha, from up the street, was on the porch. She asked Tammy why we were being so mean and putting Carol in a nursing home. Tammy told her that she needed to mind her own business. She told Martha that she did not know enough about the situation to judge it. She further told her that she was welcome to sit on the porch and talk with Carol, but she needed to keep her opinions to herself. Martha decided that it was a good idea to keep quiet.

Carol wanted to keep the paper that came about her check. She resisted Tammy having the paper. It was hers, she said. Tammy told her that she needed it. She finally relented. Her check came as well, but she did not see it. We sent it right back out to the bank.

It is afternoon. The clerk at Division of Mental Health called. She is still looking for the information about Carol's doctor, psychologist, and social worker. For some unknown reason, they cannot send the papers to Eastern State Mental Hospital. I told her that I had spoken to Wayne Cook, the assistant DA, and he told me to provide the name of the doctor at the nursing home. I also told her that we had contacted the Center for Women and Children about getting a social worker for Carol. I told her that I would work with the nursing home toward getting the psychologist.

While I was on the phone with the clerk's office, Homestead Nursing called. It seems they have trouble reading the reports. They thought the report said that she had wandered into traffic several times while at Eastern State. This was not the case. When we talked to them originally, we stated that she told us she was going to get on the interstate and hitchhike back to Florida. They also had the impression that the report said she was combative. That was in the history part of the report and referred to her hitting Tammy in the shoulder. They are having the Head of Nursing call us.

Tammy is calling all the nursing homes on our list. The story is pretty much the same. There are no beds. She is going down the list in the phone book. We contacted North Point, which came highly recommended by several others. North Point told us that they had beds available. They requested that we bring her paperwork. We will stop by Homestead to gather her paperwork.

More calls. There is more explaining about Carol to complete strangers. Every call rehashes the guilt of not being able to care for her on our own. During every call, you have to reassure yourself that you are doing the right thing. This issue is not a right thing/wrong thing situation. It is an 'only thing' situation.

Every call bolsters hope. Every piece of good news builds on the last. Not everyone has room. Not everyone wants an Alzheimer's patient. Some do not accept patients with dementia. It is not a matter of rejection. It is just a matter of statistics. There is a smile in Tammy's voice.

Tammy called the Breckenridge. While they are private pay, which is not what we are looking for, they were an invaluable source of information. They recommended North Point as well. Joann even told us that she would call Cara for us. We will not abandon any other avenues, but we will concentrate more effort on this. They have beds.

Chasity, Chris, and Ian come for a visit. They are just returning from the doctor. Ian has some sort of virus. He is still growing (Kids do that). He is eleven pounds seven ounces.

Jordan is here visiting Sierra. I was kidding him about being here two days in a row. Sierra got a little snippy about it. I talked to Tammy about that. She spoke to Sierra. Sierra asked to speak to me. She apologized to me. I apologized to her. It seems that all of this is wearing more heavily than I realized. I need to make a much greater effort to keep the water in the tub.

We drove to Homestead and picked up the papers from Eastern State. From there, we went to North Point. Tammy talked to Cara. She showed Tammy around the place and talked with her about Carol. She is taking this to the review board in the morning. She is optimistic that they will be able to accept Carol. Tammy is crossing her fingers and toes.

Before we got back, Chelsea called. It seems Carol is on the porch crying about Jim Young, and her furniture, and her Momma. She says she cannot take it. We were just a few minutes from being home. It is hard to take Carol with us to certain places. It is even more difficult to leave her at home with the kids. Once we were home, she was calm. She lay on the couch and napped for a bit. I noticed that she does not turn on the light when she goes to the bathroom. I think she does not remember where the light switch is located.

There is trouble on the porch. Our new neighbor picked Sierra up and squeezed her. She asked him to put her down. He did not until she asked a second time. It hurt her stomach. While, I am sure he meant no harm, there is no reason for a thirty-three year old man to wrestle with a fifteen-year-old girl. He has just left for Frankfort. We will talk to him when he returns. Life goes on.

The evening is progressing. The kids are outside playing, except for Kyle, who is grounded. Tasha is stopping by to pay for the mattress and box springs she bought from my daughter. We are donating sheets. Donavon is outside with the kids. Kyle George mowed the yard for me. I surprised him with ten dollars. He was figuring it was a freebie. He had volunteered to do it when we moved in nine months ago.

Donavon is in and panting. Carol asks if she should get him some water. I assured her that he knew where his water dish was located. Probably less than a minute passed when he panted again. Again, she asked if he needed water. Once more, I told her that he had water in his dish and he knew where it was. A few minutes later, he was panting again. She got up from the couch, saying that she was going to get him some water. For the third time, I told her that he had water. Third time was a charm. She got the message, for now.

As I said earlier, I never knew the Carol that was head bookkeeper for a sub contractor at the Kennedy Space Center. I never met the Carol that started her own salvage company and ran it for years. This is the only Carol I have known. Still, it is frustrating to know how this disease has ravaged her mind. It is painful to see how her thought processes have become scattered. When she is arguing about some fact in this process, she likes to say, "How would you feel if it were you?" I cannot imagine. I cannot fathom how it must be. There are times that she knows she is bad off. In those moments, she too is frustrated by her spotted memory.

In a conversation earlier today, they were talking about Sierra's birthday. She was born the day after Christmas. Carol said, talking to Sierra, "you were? I didn't know that." This nearly broke Tammy's heart. She tries to be so strong about all this. She will tell you, if you ask, that she has no choice. She will do what has to be done. She will make the decisions that no one else is willing to make. She will go the miles that no one wants to travel. When she is finished and this is completed, she will gather the broken pieces of her heart and finally take time to heal. She does not have time to do that today. Every night and several times during the day, Tammy will go to her hiding place. I will wrap that hiding place around her. She will find her comfort in my arms. I will try to be there to hold her, always.

It is ten-forty five PM. That is several hours before our normal bedtime during this. We are going to finish a few chores and sneak off to bed early. The last thing of the day is to call my parents. I want them to pray about North Point.

Good night all.

Friday, June 4th

Tammy is off on her morning run. She has taken Kyle to school. She has an appointment with Dr. Einbecker this morning. They moved her appt. up to give them the afternoon off. This was fine with us.

Tammy is back from the doctor with no better news than ever. He does want her to wear her TENS unit all the time. We are going to make a trip to the grocery before the visit. We are going to do this alone. We need the time.

When we returned from the grocery, we discovered the trashcans without bags. Carol has taken out the trash. Part of the problem with this is that she will take it out before the cans are half filled. Once more, I reminded her about the kid's chores. She ignored Chella telling her this. I think Chella has reached her patience limit with Carol. She also put a bowl of water in the middle of the living room floor. Tammy nearly tripped over it.

Cara came for the home visit around two-thirty. She was very pleasant. She talked to Carol about the nursing home. They chatted while Carol jumped from subject to subject. Overall, it went well. It went well enough that Cara is going to recommend to her board that they accept Carol for placement. This is a good thing. Tammy is teary. There are parts of this that are will never be easy. Even though this is what is best, even though this is what is necessary, it is not easy. Sometimes, doing the right thing is the most difficult. Somewhere in the back of our minds, we have this idea that if it is the right thing, it will be simple. It just isn't so.

Dealing with Carol is a daylong thing. Some days it is a long daylong thing. Tammy has talked Carol into another shower. This time she insisted on Carol washing her hair. She took her shower and muttered all the time she was doing it. She talks all the time. When she is not talking to us, she is talking to the dog, or to herself. The most curious thing about it is that I think she thinks the dog is going to answer her. If the dog does answer her, I am going to North Point.

Looks like Jordan is headed our way. I guess we are staying home this evening. We try to get out with our friends on Fridays to have some adult conversation. We like to enjoy some adult laughs. This is becoming increasingly harder to do. Sierra is best at handling Carol. She handles her as she does the kids that she baby-sits. She has sternness in her voice and Carol responds to that. The same is true with Tammy and I. Chelsea has a softer voice. Carol can ignore her.

Saturday, June 5th

We took Carol and Kyle with us this morning to Mom and Dad's house. On the trip over, we had the windows down in the Blazer. Carol fussed about her 'head blowing off' and tried to convince Kyle to put up his window. When he refused, she got snippy with him. Tammy scolded her about it. She fussed for about five minutes about it. She moves from one extreme to the other. Kyle is either the cutest thing or the rudest thing.

When we left, she again fussed about her hair blowing. She put her window up and Tammy gave her a brush to fix her hair. We drove about two blocks and she was asking how she could put her window down. Tammy told her that if she put it down it would blow her hair. She said she was not worried about her hair blowing. This is how it is constantly.

On our way home, we passed many yard sales. Tammy loves yard sales. She, Kyle, and Carol are going back out to do some shopping. I gave Carol ten dollars to have herself to spend at the yard sales. She cried. I know she hates being dependant. She hates the feeling that she has lost her independence. This disease is a thief. Worse than that, it is a thief without conscience. It is mindless of the devastation it leaves in its wake. It is the silent enemy.

During the yard sale adventure, Carol broke down twice. She lost her money. She had put it in her eyeglass case and could not find it.

She was frantic. Tammy found it for her. Within ten seconds, she had lost it again. Tammy decided it was best if she kept the money. Carol agreed. The simplest of trips becomes complicated. Complicated trips become impossible. She has no sense of decorum. If she sees a heavy person, she will loudly comment, "That's a fat one". If she sees blacks, she will, just as loudly, comment, "There are lots of niggers here". As you can guess, going anywhere that you will encounter other people is difficult.

Today, while visiting the various yard sales, they passed a truck with a man waiting for his wife. He was large and black. Carol said, "That's a big black nigger. He's black as the ace of spades." Tammy stopped her and told her that was not acceptable. Carol said she did not mean it that way. Tammy told her that she <u>did</u> mean it that way.

It was not five minutes later she was talking about a 'fat' woman at the next yard sale. She asked Tammy who that fat girl was that was at our house on Friday. She also asked if she were a dyke. Tammy told her that the girl had a name. She was not 'that fat girl'. Tammy told her that we have a variety of friends in all manners of shapes, sizes, colors, and sexual orientations. She tried to explain to Carol that those words hurt people. She understands for five minutes.

Tomorrow, we will be hosting a picnic with one of the internet groups to which we belong. We have no choice but to take Carol with us. We hope she will sit quietly at a picnic table. We will not tolerate her berating our friends. She will have to understand this. We will also be going to church in the morning. The same rules will apply.

Evening

Chelsea bought Tammy a video tape. It was the movie, The Truman Show. We are watching it now, with Carol's running commentary on everything that happens in it. The first night that we have absolutely alone is going to be sweet. The kids are going to Florida with their dad for a month. They are leaving on Tuesday, if all goes according to plan. Carol will be in the nursing home by Tuesday evening, if all goes according to plan. Tuesday evening is going to be a cuddle on the couch watching movies night. We will hide out from the computer and the phone. Being incommunicado sounds perfect.

Supper is served. Carol raved about the food. Of course, we are going to get her fat, she says. She finished her supper and took her plate to the kitchen. As usual, we had to remind her not to do the dishes. Kyle was in the kitchen eating and reading some refrigerator magnet. Carol called him a jackass, for some unknown reason. We told him to ignore it. The situation is wearing everyone thin.

You can read all the books there are on the subject. There are symptom lists from here to yon. For all the preparations you can make, every case is different. There is nothing we read that prepared us for the sheer magnitude of this. I understand the sympathy expressed by others that have been here. When this is behind us, we will express the same sympathies to others starting their journey. In my mind, I know they will be polite. They will accept our sympathies. Their case will be different. Theirs will be the smooth one. I know. I thought the same thing.

Sunday, June 6th

Today is picnic day. We spent the morning getting the last of the supplies. Well, it was late morning to early afternoon when we started. Carol is excited. By two PM, we are ready to head to the park. We are taking both vehicles. There are eight of us going from here. It was an interesting trip to the park. About a mile or so from the house, the brakes on Tammy's car start giving out. We pull over to check. She is low on brake fluid. She has to pump them brakes to keep them working. We decide to continue.

A couple miles later, Tammy calls my cell phone. She has had a blow out. I still have to get to the park to set up as we have over forty people on their way there. She is going to find a place to pull over. I called my brother-in-law to pick her up. He lives near where she stopped. Turns out, it was not flat. It had separated. We thought her spare was flat. Turns out, it was not. Bobby changed her tire and they were on their way.

I was at the park and set up when she finally got there. The picnic was great. There were about forty - fifty people there. Carol had a great time. She flirted with Jeff, a thirty-nine year old. He enjoyed talking to her. He even asked if he could visit her once she was settled into a nursing home. She talked about him only on the trip home. The weather was great. The food was good. The company was fine. It felt great to get out and mingle. It felt good to be grown-ups.

It was seventy-six degrees out today. It was a beautiful day. Evening is settling in and the temperature has dropped to seventy-three degrees. Carol is going on about how cold it has gotten. "That temperature is dropping out there", she says repeatedly. She cannot believe how chilly it is. I checked the weather and told her it had dropped three degrees. She was happy.

Monday, June 7th

It is nine-thirty AM. Carol is out of bed. Kyle is at school. Tammy has just lain back down. She did not sleep very well last night because of pain. Carol took her cup of coffee out to the porch. She loves sitting on the porch drinking her morning coffee. She was not out there very long, before she came back in complaining about how insufferable the heat was. She just cannot understand how it got so hot out there. I checked the temperature. It is sixty-seven degrees. That is six degrees colder than last night when she was complaining about how cold it was.

I need to find a doctor today to give Carol a physical. She has to have one before she goes into the nursing home. Today we find out the decision of North Point. If it is a yes, we want to move quickly as not to lose an available bed. We also want to move on the effort to move Mary here. Medicaid of Florida will pay for ambulance transport to Kentucky. We are not sure what arrangements would have to be made to bring her belongings.

There are constantly things to remind her. She does not ever remember to leave the bathroom door open. This morning I caught her trying to feed the dog potato chips. I reminded her that we do not feed the dog people food. She could not see me seeing her. She had the chip at the dog's mouth. When I spoke, she jerked the chip away, and said, "I'm not". It is rather obvious that she has been. Whenever there is food out, he runs right to Carol.

Tammy was just in the kitchen. There is water all over the table. She said that she did not know how all this water got on there. Carol told her that the fridge was leaking. She became very defensive about it. Tammy told her that she was not buying the fridge leaking on the table. Carol went directly to pity. She has so much on her mind. She is worried about so many things. I checked while Tammy was walking Donavon. There was a large cup on the table with melted ice and some residual soda in it. When Carol was getting the chips that she tried to feed to the dog, she knocked it over.

Phone is ringing. It is Cara from North Point. The board at the nursing home had some questions. They were about bathing, showering, getting in and out of chairs, and assistance walking. She can bath herself, if reminded to do so. She can get in and out of chairs unassisted. She walks well for a seventy-two year old with arthritis in her knees. Cara said she would get in touch with us later today.

Cara called back. They are ready to accept Carol. We are taking her for a tour this afternoon. Carol is confused. She does not know what is going on, even though she has been informed all along the way. She is talking about Florida and calling it Lexington. She still does not understand her need for helped. She is telling Tammy that she did not even know her five years ago when Dr. Idiculla told her that Carol had Alzheimer's disease.

We have drifted into the Carol zone. It is like a frog jumping from one lily pad to another. We are the second frog in the pond trying to keep up. We are in Jim Young town, and discussing furniture. Now she has a heart problem. Most of the time she tells us that she has no health problems. She does not remember Eastern State Mental Hospital. She has been away from there two weeks. She swears that she saw Raymond Young at the bottom of the hill. She has not seen him for many years. She thinks she has talked to Jim Young and he wants her to come back to Florida. Jump jump jump. When all the jumping is finished, we are on the same lily pad, and Carol does not remember moving off the original pad. Everyone is exhausted and nothing gained.

The mail has run. There were a few pieces concerning Carol. I opened them. There was a bank statement and some papers from Medicare about some doctor visits Carol had in April. There was a minor problem in the laundry room. I fixed that. When I returned, the papers for Carol were gone from the coffee table. I picked up the envelopes. They were empty. Carol got defensive when I told Tammy they were missing.

I looked around the room, thinking I might have moved them. They were nowhere to be found. All the while, Carol is going on about how she did not touch anything. I walked out to the porch and there they were, in Carol's purse. Forgetful or not, she is sneaky. She will tell you she understands we are handling her affairs now. Then, she will turn around and demand to have any mail addressed to her. I am not sure the word 'exasperating' covers this. These papers were trivial. They had no bearing on anything we are working with. The problem will be when she thieves something that is important. She may horde away some vital document. "That is my business", she will say. It is one of her favorite catch phrases when she cannot remember about what she is arguing.

It is later in the afternoon now. Carol has calmed down a bit. One of her worries was the condition of Grammy. We have called Rockledge Health and Rehab to check on her. In a conversation with Douglas, the director, we found out that Fred Oliver had visited Grammy. That is an interesting piece of news. It seems that Fred was a cardiologist or head of veterinary medicine at a hospital in Lexington depending on who is telling at one time. He got involved in drugs. The last anyone heard he was working as a bagboy at a grocery. We are setting the wheels in motion to move Grammy to Lexington.

I have made a discovery. It is more like an analogy, actually. We all have a junk drawer in our home somewhere. It is where things go that have no specific place to be. When we need something and cannot find it anywhere. We go to the junk drawer. Somewhere in there lies the hope of finding it. We saw it once. It could not disappear. Therefore, we pilfer through the drawer in our quest.

Carol's mind is like this. There is one difference. Everything in her life is now in this drawer. When she tries to find the right facts for any given situation, she has to search through the entire drawer. I remember dad sending me to find a bolt for something he was trying to fix. I would open that drawer and there would be what seemed like a million various sized screws. I would take a stick and start digging. I swear, sometimes I can hear that digging sound when Carol is trying to remember something she knew yesterday.

Monday afternoon

We are taking Carol to North Point for her tour. During the drive, she asked us when the mail runs. She told us she was expecting a letter. I asked her whom the letter was to be from and I would look for it. She said it was just from a friend. Tammy told her to come off it. She told her that we knew she took the letters and put them in her purse. We told her that we had removed them. She admitted she knew that the mail had come.

It is just after four-thirty. We have just returned from taking Carol on a tour of North Point. She liked the facility. It is impressive. We are taking her back tomorrow at eleven AM and she will stay there. They are admitting her 'Medicaid pending'. We stopped at the Medicaid office on our way home to make an appointment. She has to have Nursing Home Medicaid, which is different from regular Medicaid. My head spins. There is elder care Medicaid, regular Medicaid, children's Medicaid, pregnancy Medicaid, nursing home Medicaid, and still other Medicaid's. Mrs. Roach set up an appointment for June twenty-ninth. She said she would approve her on that date. She also told us that Medicare would pay for the first twenty-one days. I have breathed a tentative sigh. Tammy is reserving her sigh until tomorrow. I can see a light at the end of the tunnel. I hope it is not the train.

I think we have contact Alzheimer. It is kind of like a contact buzz. We are tired a lot and forget things easily. We are hoping this will pass quickly. If it does not, however, we will not remember it.

Ronnie called. He is on his way. He is taking the kids to Florida for a month. Sometime within the next forty-eight hours, the house will belong to us again. There will be a lot of crying and sighing then. We have decided that the first night will be 'no explanations' night. There will be no explaining of the rules to the kids. There will be no explaining of everything to Carol. There will be quiet. There will be snuggling on the couch. There will be movies without talking. There will be uninterrupted reading. Did I mention there would be snuggling? There are so many things that we took for granted. I am sure we will be taking them for granted again soon enough, but for about two weeks, we will cherish it. We will cook small, if we can figure out how to do that.

Kayla just ran in to tell us that Carol was walking off and Chelsea could not stop her. Sierra went to take care of it. She got Carol back on the porch. Carol was walking up the sidewalk toward Limestone Street. She came in the house fussing about the girls fussing at her.

She said she had a note of things she wanted to remember tomorrow when she was at the nursing home. I asked her if she minded showing it to me. She pulled it out and proceeded to read it to me. She mentioned that it had Jim Young's name on it, but it was there from months ago. I read it. She wrote it on an envelope that I gave her this morning. There was Jim's cell phone number on it. There was a note to Jim telling him not to come to this state. Earlier, she tried to tell Chelsea that we Okayed her using the phone. Chelsea did not buy that. She also asked Sierra if she could use her cell phone. Sierra told her that she could not.

She sat and fussed about her life. She fussed about not being able to go next door. Once we gathered the evidence and listened to her denials, it was obvious what she was trying to do. She was trying to find a way to call Jim. She tried to convince me that she helped Martha move out. The only snag in that was that Martha moved yesterday and we were at the picnic. She insists she helped Martha move her dishes. This must be lily pad #212.

Evening

Carol is still yammering on about the same old stuff. Tammy is reading to Kyle at bedtime. He and the kids are leaving tomorrow for a month away. Carol's constant fussing has grated on everyone's nerves. We are all able to go from zero to bitchy real quick.

Carol thinks she has spoke to Jim three times since she has been here. She further thinks she has to get her furniture out of the house by Friday of this week, because Jim told her he was moving. This was in one of the three conversations she had with him this week. Carol cannot use the phones here. The house phone is mostly hidden. We all carry our cell phones with us ninety percent of the time. The few times they are not with us, she would not be able to find them, nor would she know how to unlock them.

She goes on and on about the same old subjects with an "I would be better off dead" tossed in there every now and then. It does get old. The effect is so subtle that you do not even know it is there until you are suddenly full and overflowing. As much as this is about Carol, it is also about me. This requires a different kind of patience. You can be patient with a child. They are learning. It is an unrelated dynamic with Carol. She is not learning. She is un-learning. As many times as we explain is as many times as she is going to forget. Getting angry with her is useless. She will not remember it in fifteen minutes either. She is going to remember it the same way she asks before you clarify it.

This is the heartbreak of this disease. Nothing you do is going to make a difference. You kindness will be forgotten. Your anger will be lost. The way you treat an Alzheimer's patient is for your peace of mind. It is about doing everything you can and living with that effort. Sometimes it is about getting it outside of you. It needs expressing, even though it will be forgotten. It is an emotional roller coaster ride. I am not a psychologist. I am not a counselor. I am a student of the human heart and emotion. This is just what I see.

I know this much. I sleep at night. My advice works for me. It might work for you. It might not. In all of this writing, I have sought to show you just how individual this ordeal will be. It will not end tomorrow when Carol is safe in a good facility. As bad as she is, she is going to get worse. She will not only forget the events of today, she will forget years. She will forget parents. She will forget her children. Can you imagine this? Pick any day about which I have written. Now, imagine that it is the best day she is going to have for the rest of her life. She may rally from time to time. With the aid of medicines, she may gain some lucidity. She is still, however, on a downhill ride.

Prepare yourself for the most heart-wrenching ride of your life. It will be worse than you can imagine. I am not the same man I was a month ago. Alzheimer's disease has changed me. I hope it has changed me for the better. Time will tell.

It is eleven-thirty in the evening. Carol has just begun her pocketbook search. Tammy gave her a larger pocketbook. It is on the floor against the wall. It is still unused, even though she was thrilled when she got it. It is just one more forgotten thing.

Tammy is cleaning up a few messes in the fridge. Carol left a partially eaten bowl of potato salad with crackers in there. Tammy did not say a word about what it was. She just said something about someone leaving something gross in the fridge. Carol immediately began denying it could be her. "I haven't even been in the fridge today. I have not even been by it except one time. I walked by it", she said. She left a partially eaten cooked hamburger patty in the door of the fridge. She adamantly denied it was she. The thing is, no one was saying it was anyone. She is like a child. She knows she did it, and yet denies it. This is just what we need, a seventy-two year old seven year old.

It is time for Tammy and me to relax our brains with some online word games.

Tuesday, June 8th

Today is going to be the most difficult day since this began. There are several reasons for this. Today is the actual last day of school for Kyle. There is an award presentation program commencing at one PM. Carol is being admitted to the nursing home this morning. Then, sometime this afternoon, Tammy's ex, Ronnie is taking the

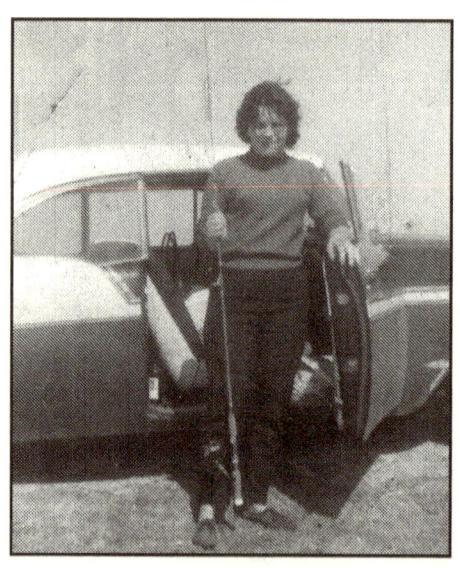

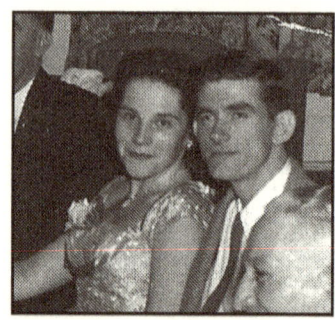

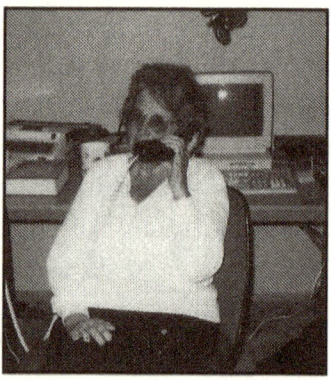

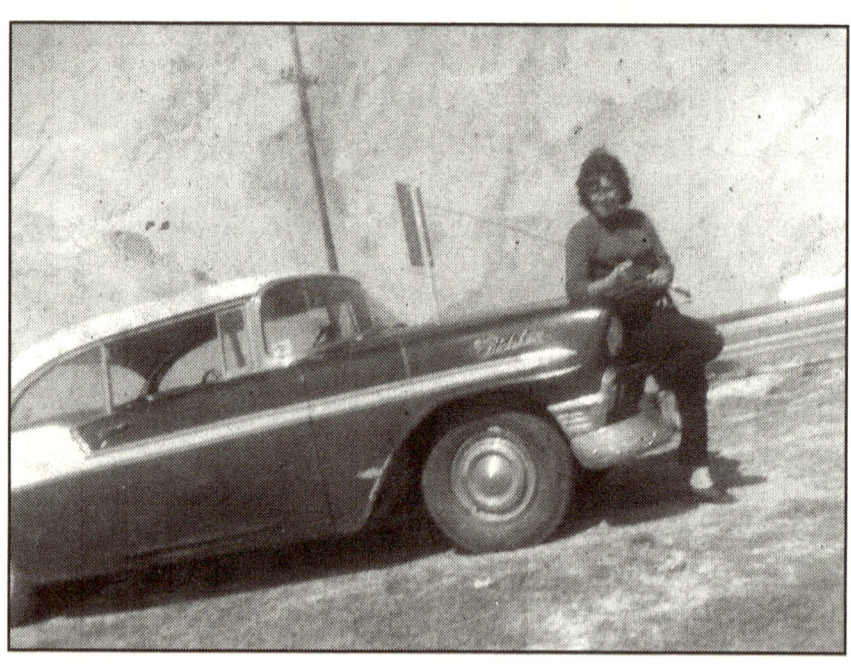

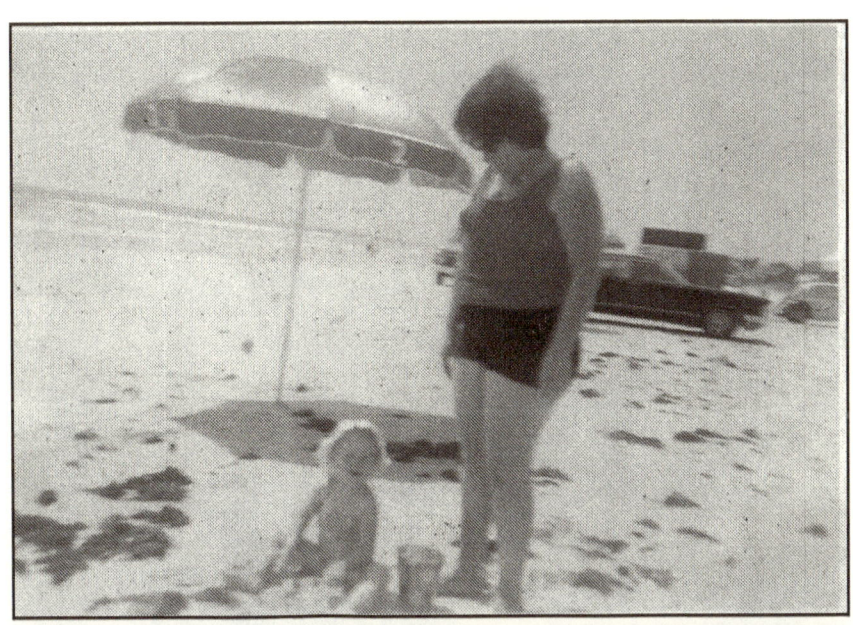

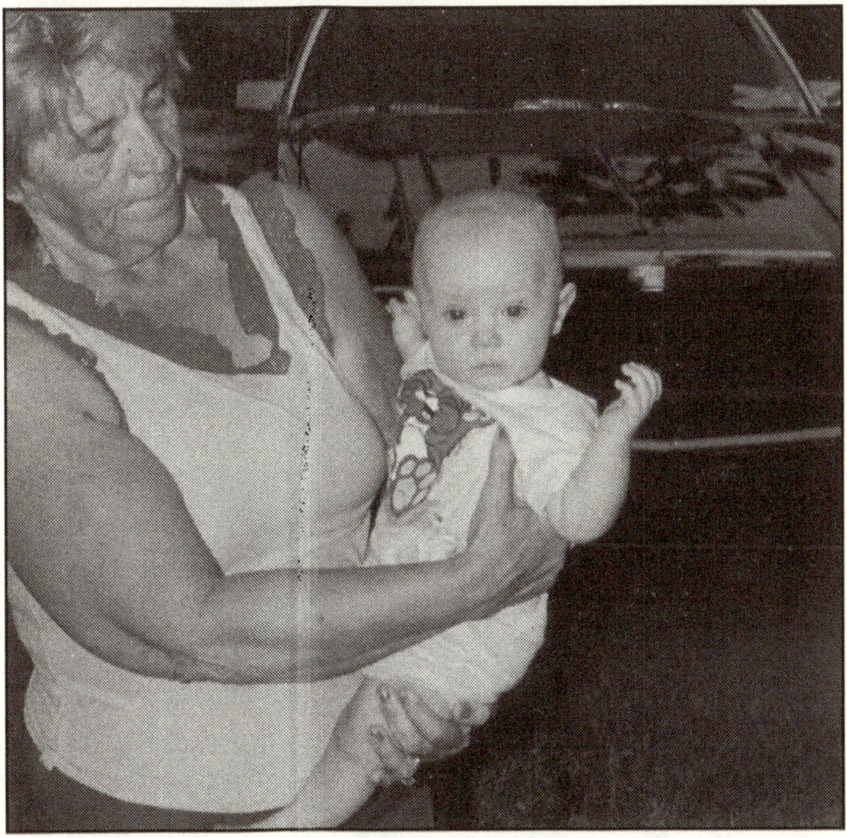

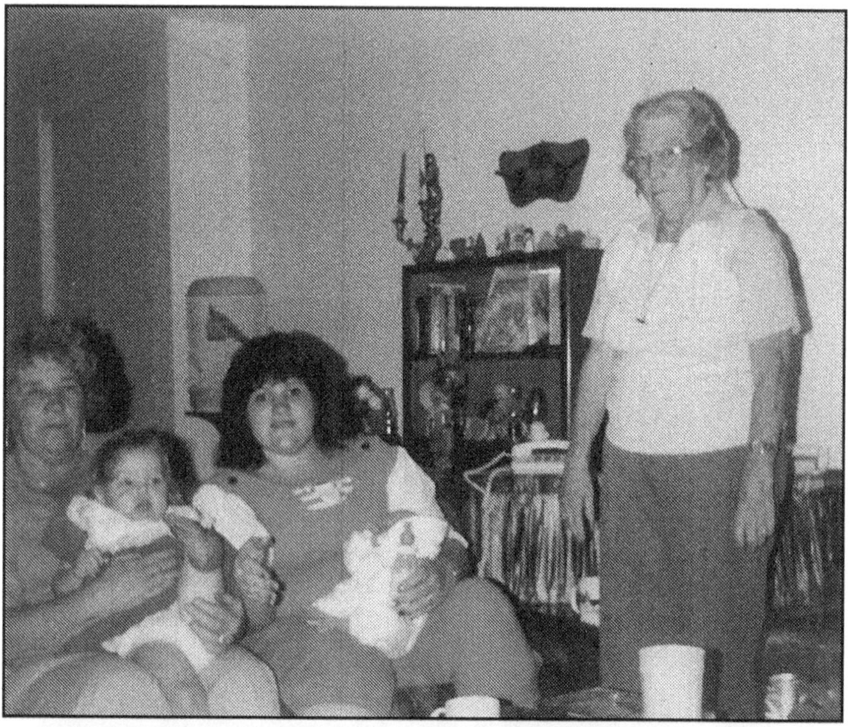

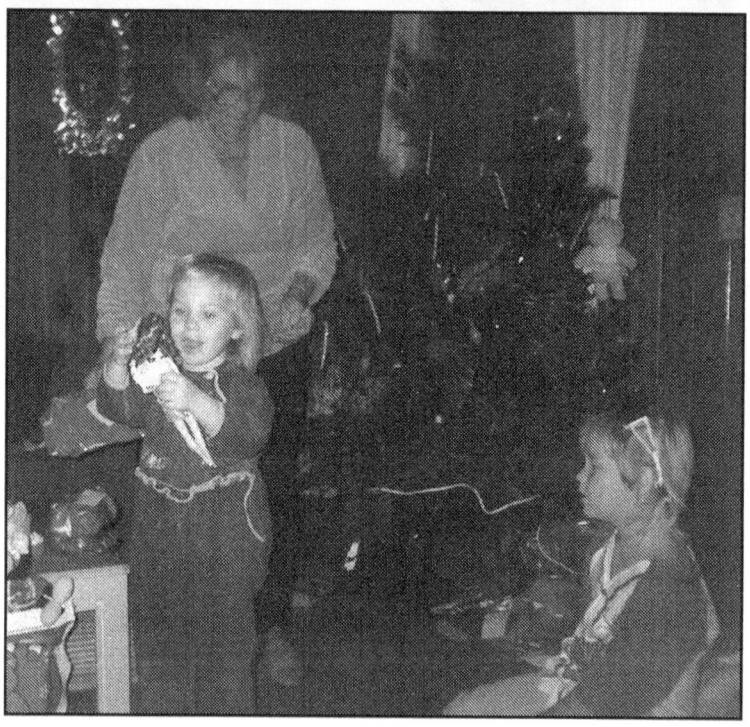

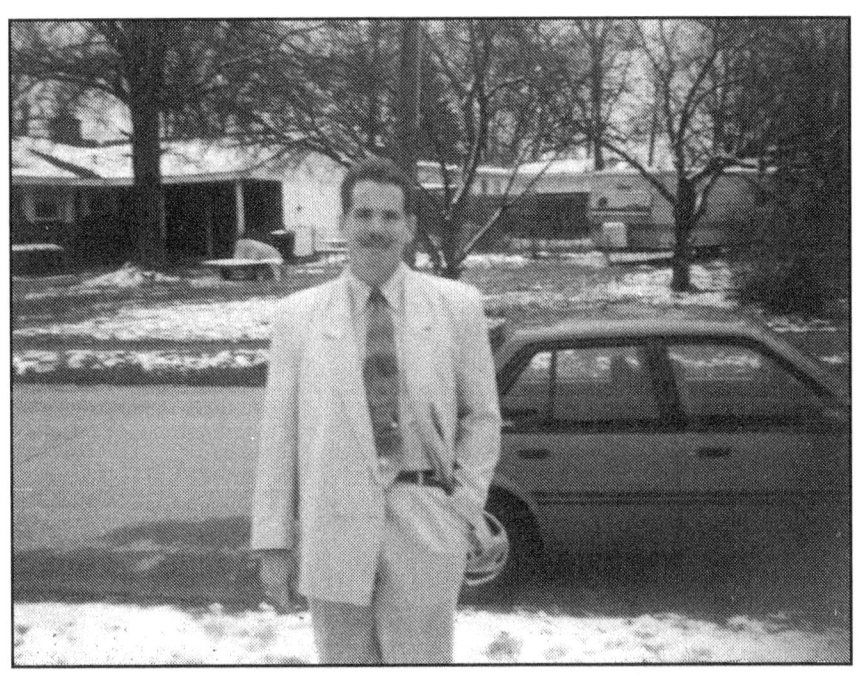

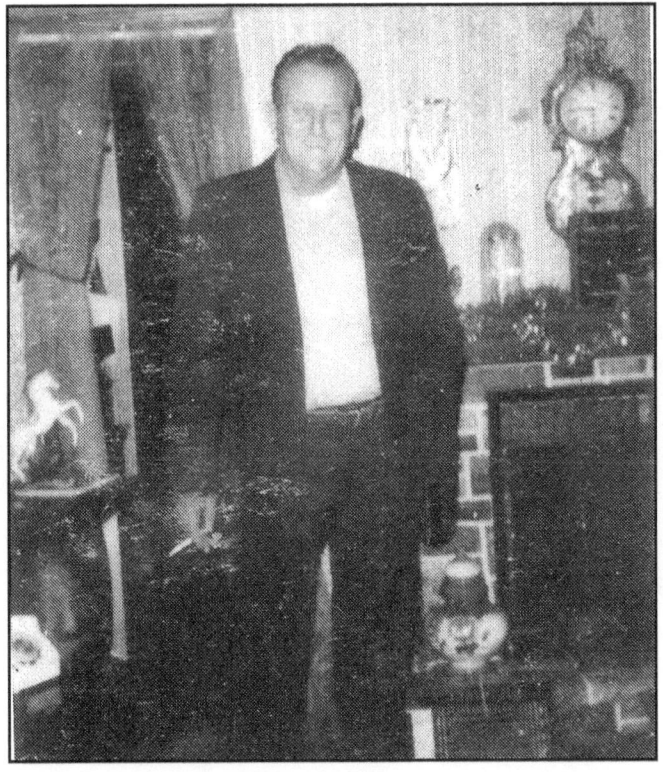

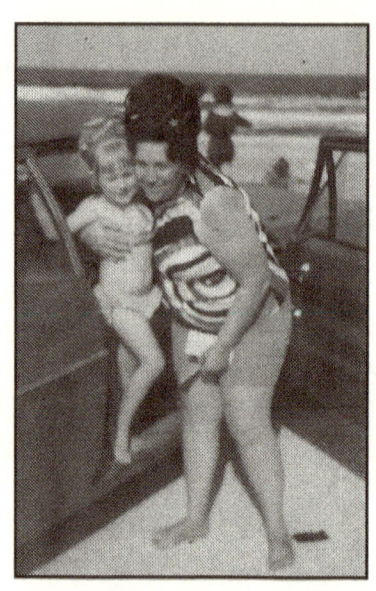

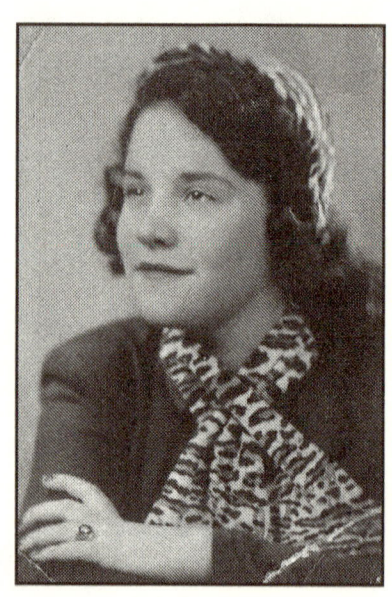

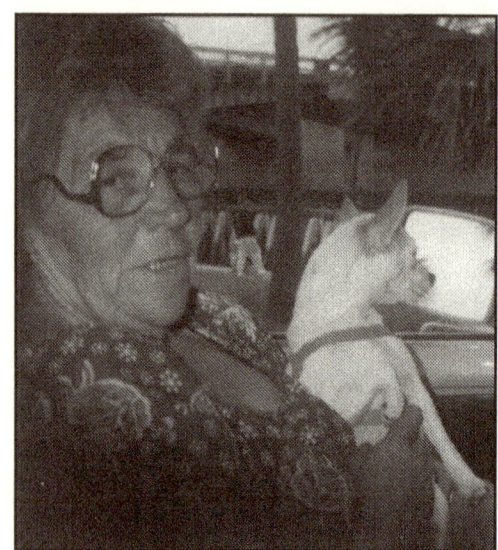

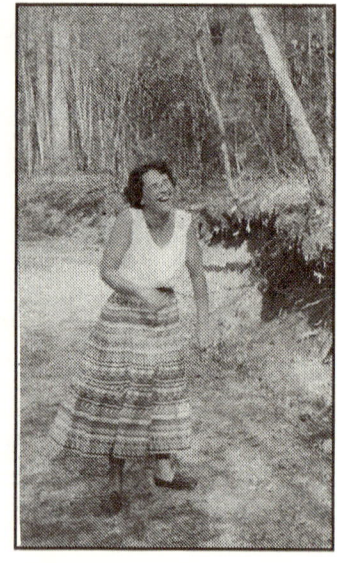

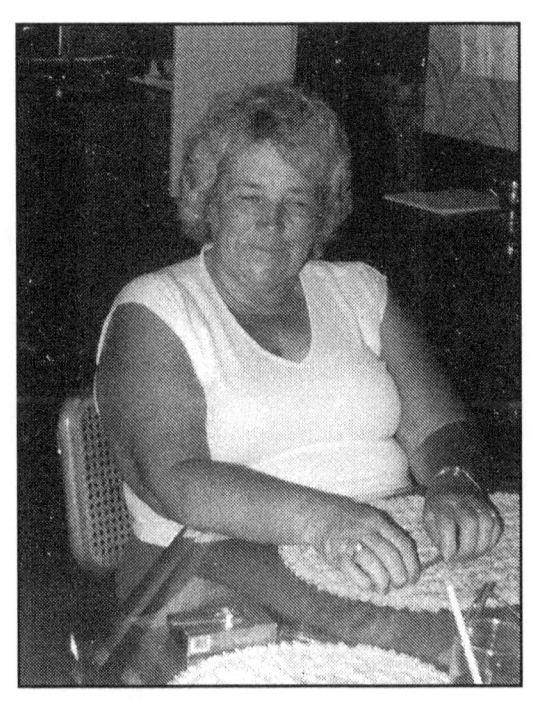

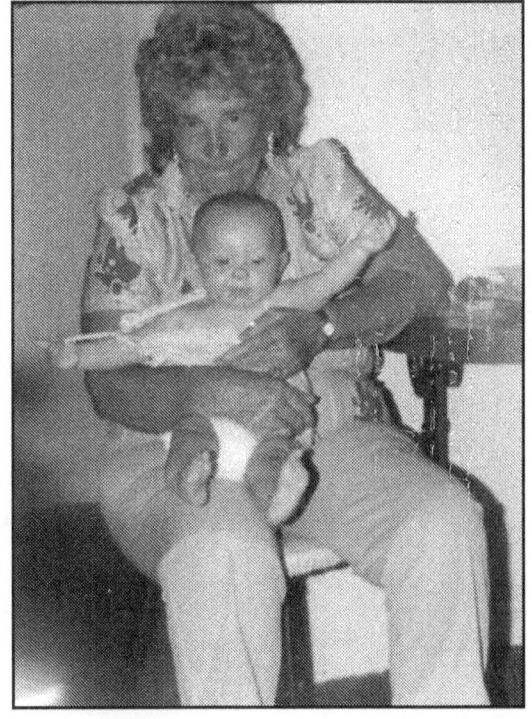

kids to Florida for a month. All of this is culminating into one whirlwind of a day.

Tammy is up and going after 'just one more minute of the chest'. She has Kyle awake and dressed for school. Sierra is awake and ready. Carol is ready to go as well. They will take Kyle to school and then go to physical therapy for Tammy's wrist. Tammy called me about a quarter before nine. The physical therapy office was not open. There were several patients waiting. She decided to leave. Waiting is never a good plan when you have Carol onboard.

Tammy made a few stops on her way back home. Once home, she gave her Mom clothes to wear. She and I got dressed as well. We dressed for the awards ceremony. Carol decided to try to discuss her way out of going to the nursing home. She reiterated that she had to go to Florida to get her belongings. She cannot do that if she is in the nursing home. I told her once again that she is not going to Florida when we go. I made it simple. We will not have room. Just as we were about to leave, she decided that what she was wearing was too hot. She needed to change clothes. She was half undressed by the time I stopped her. I told her that all her clothes were packed. There was nothing for her to change into. She fussed and fussed. I told her that I would take her in her bra if she did not get dressed. She complied. She tried to say that this trip was going to be for checking out the nursing home. We have told her that she will be there for at least one month as a trial basis. Unless there are problems with the nursing home, she is where she will live.

We made sure that we could take her home with us for overnight visits before we agreed to allow her to stay. We made sure that everyone could visit. North Point even told us that we could bring the dog to visit her.

Once there, she wanted to make sure that Cara knew this was just a temporary stay. When the nurse interviewed her for their files, she again pointed out that it was just temporary. Her roommate's name is Mary. Mary's daughter-in-law is one of the workers on that section. While Tammy was filling out papers with Cara, Carol and I sat in the cafeteria area. Ollie, the floor nurse, interviewed us there.

Anyone that stopped and talked to us for more than five minutes got the 'only temporary' speech.

We made a list of all Carol's clothes and belongings for North Point. They keep up with all of that. They are having a new chiller installed for the air conditioning unit, so it is warm there today. We will be there tomorrow to bring Carol a fan. We will open her escrow account there at that time. Her money will remain there and she can use it for trips to the beauty salon and other organized functions.

As we were leaving, she tried to whittle the length of the stay down to ten days. Yesterday it was a thirty-day stay. This morning it was a twenty-day stay. The irony of it all is that we could agree to it being a ten-day stay, and she would not remember it tomorrow.

Driving down the road, I asked Tammy if she was ready to breathe that sigh yet. It still is not easy. It will get easier. It will not be tomorrow. It will not be the day after either. Eventually, Carol will settle in. Eventually, we will get Grammy in. Someday this will be easier. We will look back on this and appreciate it for what it is. It is a difficult time in Carol's life and we were there for her. When others walked away, we walked up. As I said previously, this is not about how noble we are. It is not about our goodness. It is just about family. It is about taking care of your own. It is about doing the best you can with what you have. Today, it is about getting through today.

One very interesting fact came through Tammy's talk with Cara while signing papers. It seems that we did not need to be Carol's legal guardian to get her into a nursing home. As her next of kin, Tammy could have been working on the nursing home part from the beginning. With Carol's signature, we could have done most of the things we have done. The guardianship is legal, however, and that is necessary for some aspects of this. It might have been easier, mentally, to do all this if Carol were already provided for.

One PM

We were in the Johnson Elementary gym for the presentation of awards. Kyle received his Primary Citizenship award, his Math MVP award, his reading award, and a school jacket. Ronnie, Linda, and

Chris (Tammy's oldest son) arrived in time to see Kyle receive all his awards. It was a great time.

We came home, where the kids are making final preparation for their trip. I said my goodbyes to each one privately. I did not want to bother Ronnie. He has some residual issues about his kids loving me. I do not have these issues, but I will not inflame them in him. Tammy is pre-tearing. It is going to be difficult for her. Part of her relationship with them is a daily interaction. Her love and their love will not diminish during this trip, but that physical contact will be missing.

Tammy's uncle, Fred, called today. She has not heard from him in years. Fred is Carol's brother. Tammy caught him up on all the news. She asked if he wanted to intercede for Grammy as her guardian. He told her that she seemed to be doing a fine job of it. We do not look for much help here. It is something to which we have become accustomed. It was one month ago, May 8th, that Jim Young drove away back to Florida. It was one month ago that various relatives told us that they would be there to help. We have not seen hide or hair of any one of them since. If you are reading this on the front end of your ordeal, I cannot stress loudly enough, be prepared to do this alone. Accept the help of strangers. They may be the only offers you get.

Evening

We rented a few movies and settled in for the evening. The kids are with Ronnie. Carol is safe at North Point. We tried not to answer the phone when it rang. That did not work. It rang one time. It was Leonard, a friend and co-worker of Tammy's. The conversation was short. We went back to uninterrupted movie watching.

Wednesday, June 9th

We slept in. There were not kids to wake and no one to watch. It was around ten AM before we both made it out of bed. Tammy went to physical therapy at eleven AM. She called me around noon to say she was on her way home. There were matters we needed to take care of. Therefore, we set about doing that.

While we were out, North Point called to ask us to come there. Carol had packed her suitcase. She cussed the staff. She called them names. Then, she told them her husband was coming to pick her up. We were going there to take Carol a fan later. We made it early. When we arrived, Jeanie and Bonnie were downstairs with another patient. They told us she was dressed up pretty. Her suitcase was packed.

Upstairs, we found Carol with one of the counselors. He told us the 'temperature' had dropped about thirty degrees in the last ten minutes. We took Carol outside to talk to her. She told us that her time there was up. We asked her about the reported behavior. Of course, it never happened. I could not tell if it was the dementia. It may be that we were taking a trip to Deny-ville. Carol's name could be changed to Cleopatra. She is the Queen of Denial. Nothing that happened has actually happened. Nothing in her life is ever her fault. If we just knew what she had to put up with in her life, we would understand, or so she says. We told her that her choices were here or another nursing home. Her choices did not include an idyllic country setting with a little house for her and Grammy. They did not include living with us. They did not include going back to Florida to Jim Young.

Tammy took her suitcase back to the room and unpacked it. I talked to Carol in the courtyard. Tammy is struggling hard with this. She has great internal resentment for the hell she went through as a child. Tammy and I talked about emotional scarring. She told me these were not scars. They were still open wounds. They have never healed. Now, with Carol in the shape she is in, there is no hope for closure. It kills her inside. Add to that, that every time we tell Carol she has to stay in the nursing home, she claims we do not love her, and it gets even worse.

We talked to the staff and director at North Point. They assured us they were not 'kicking her out'. They figure it will take a week or two for Carol to settle in. This behavior is more about the change than anything else. We gave the staff, counselor, and director some ideas to help. Carol is obsessive about cleaning. When she fusses, they are going to ask her to help them clean. They are going to give her washcloths to fold. They are going to let her dust things. This will distract her from whatever she thinks needs to be fussed about. She cannot hold both thoughts at the same time. She will clean and forget the second. At least, that is our hope. It has worked at home.

This was a break for Tammy. Inside, she does not want to come back to visit. She wants to forget she has a mother. She wants to forget she has a father. The problem with all of that is that it is not in her to do either. It is not in her emotional makeup to walk away. This battle rages inside of her. My part is to support her. If she is wrong, I tell her. If she is right, I tell her. I will support her either way. I will love her enough to cover any gap.

Other than this, our honeymoon/vacation is progressing well. Time alone will heal this. We will see what this evening brings. We will see what tomorrow will bring.

Another evening to us is working. We enjoyed a movie, snuggled on the couch. Tammy says it is starting to feel way too good. It is a great manner to relax. With the exception of the time we were at North Point this afternoon, there were no long bouts of explaining.

Thursday, June 10th

Chasity went to the Emergency Room last night for a urinary tract infection. She did not go to work today; therefore, she did not bring Ian at seven AM. I was up at seven anyway. I stayed up for a bit and then went back to bed. We got up around ten AM, again. The kids are safe in Florida.

Tammy went to physical therapy around eleven AM. I made a trip to the union hall to pick up papers necessary for a court matter. We were both back home by noon. There were no calls on the phone from North Point. This is a good thing. We will visit Carol this afternoon.

Tammy and I decided to go out for lunch prior to visiting Carol. It was great to sit and talk without interruption. We talked about politics. We talked about presidents of the past. It was adult conversation; sweet, wonderful, adult conversation. I did find out some interesting news. It seems that Carol was married after her divorce to Jim. In her mind, she thinks it was to Jim again, but it was not. It was to Jim's cousin, John. He was a veteran. She took care of him until he died. She may be entitled to some Veteran's benefits. We will begin that search when we get home.

Late afternoon

We just returned from North Point. This was a good visit. Carol was playing Bingo. We talked to the nursing staff about ways to distract Carol when she begins to fuss. Give her a dust rag. Give her a broom. She will lose track of the reason she was fussing in the first place.

They are moving Carol to the Amelia ward. It is just for Alzheimer's patients. She has tried to get on the elevator a few times. The patients wear armbands that have a sensor module on them. If they go out certain doors, it sets off an alarm. It also shuts down the elevator.

Carol was much calmer. We discussed the thirty-day stay. We told her about the upcoming move. Housekeeping will come in while she is out of the room and move all her belongings to the new room. They will set everything in just as it was in her old room. North Point is going to call us prior to moving Carol. We will be there to walk her over. She does not handle change well. It should help her tremendously if we are present.

The AC at North Point is finally fixed. This will help as well. It is funny; Carol complains about the heat in the day and the cold at night. The temperature seems to be an irrelevant factor.

We showed her the new clothes we brought. She wanted to discuss the thirty-day part more. We explained that the decision is not up to us. It is up to the doctor and dependant on her behavior. She assured us that she was going to behave. The medications seem to be helping. She was more cohesive today. She did not jump as much from subject to subject. Even when interrupted, she was able to regain her original thought. That is not to say that they made sense, but she was able to recall them. This was a much less frustrating visit.

Friday, June 11th

We had to be in court today on a non-related issue. This took up most of the morning. After lunch, we both lay down for a bit. This evening we attended a graduation party for three of my nieces and nephews. We did not have time to get Carol some sleeping clothes. We waited for North Point to call us about the move. They never called. It was too late to pick up the clothes or to visit and still make the party. This is the first night since she her arrival, that we have not seen her. We knew there would come a night or day, eventually, that we would not be able to visit. It does not make it any easier that it has happened. Tomorrow we will survey the aftermath.

Saturday, June 12th

I am looking out the window at the morning sunshine. The weatherman called for rain. He is still calling for it. He has moved it into afternoon to late afternoon now.

We visited Carol today. She has been moved to the Amelia ward. She does not have access to the elevators in this ward. We have to learn all new names. Tina is the activities coordinator. April is the nurse. We also met Rachel, one of the CNAs. On this ward, as the rest, the staff seems happy to be working here. This is a good thing. I told the new staff about her obsession with cleaning. I shared the dust rag technique of distraction.

She seems less manic now. The medicines seem to be helping her clarity. She still cannot remember things. Carol still thinks she talked to Jim yesterday. According to her, he called to tell her that she did not have a dog anymore. In reality, he did call us, mentioned that Docey had fleas, and was shaved and treated. We mentioned this to her. I assume this is her mind putting together how she has information about the dog while not remembering what that information is or who told her.

We visited her new room. She does not have a bed by the window now. Carol mentioned that she really liked that before, but takes this in stride. The AC is working now, so the place is much cooler. When I mentioned this to her, she told us that she had a talk with them about that and that is why they fixed it.

Carol has a basket in her room for her clothes. She keeps her clothes in it instead of the dresser. She is constantly folding and refolding these clothes. She will take a folded article of clothing out of the basket, unfold it, shake it, refold it, and lay it aside. When she has refolded the entire contents, she will put them all back in the basket, ready for the next refolding exercise.

We went to the activities room. There was a family singing gospel there. We sat in the back and talked for a bit. We left Carol there listening to the singers.

Sunday, June 13th

We went to church this morning and then out for lunch with my parents. It was a great morning. Later in the afternoon, we went to see Carol. We took her some clothes, a robe, and a purse. She told us Jeff had been to see her. She said he stayed for four to five hours. We talked to Jeff later. It was more like two to three hours. She enjoyed his visit. He listened patiently to her stories about Jim.

We took a short bio with us to put outside her door. The nursing home has a Plexiglas holder by the door to the room, for patient bios. Carol liked her bio. We met Brooklyn. She is a CNA that works Friday, Saturday, and Sunday.

Carol, Tammy, and I sat and talked about this and that. We talked about Jeff. She had trouble remembering his name. I suggested we just call him 'the cutie'. We stayed until they came for supper. We took Carol to the dining area, even though she said she had already had supper.

We were there almost an hour. That is about all Tammy can take. It is very draining on her. There are several reasons. It hurts her to see her mom in this condition. It hurts her that she is not able to care for her mom at home. As much as this hurts her, not visiting would hurt even more. It is the lesser of the two hurts. I guess it is good that not seeing her would hurt. There are one hundred fifty beds in this facility. There are over ninety patients here. We looked over the visitors log earlier while looking for Jeff's name. Each page holds about twenty names. There were less than two pages of visitors today when we left at six o'clock. I am sure there will be days when we cannot make it out, but we are going to try to be there as often as we can.

Monday, June 14th

Today was a busy day. We spent the better part of the morning going from place to place. There were many non-Carol related things to do. Life is trying to get back to our regular hectic pace. Tammy says we slowed from warp speed to merely hectic speed. It was and was not that we were so much busier. It was just that with Carol everything was complicated. I recall in my first marriage that we would go visit my wife's family in Florida on a whim. We would just jump in the car and go. Then came Audrey. Then it was make sure there are enough things for the baby. Carol is kind of like that. It is just an added degree of difficulty to everything.

Therefore, even though we were rushing about, it was still easier. Like a baby, the world had to revolve around Carol. Everything had to be about her. Everything we did, everywhere we went, in her mind, it was about her. When we spoke to one another, she always assumed it was about her. Tammy and I love talking to each other. We discuss everything from politics to the weather. This was difficult for us in that we had to talk less to each other.

We got back home late afternoon. Tammy went to see her mother alone, as my back was giving me difficulty. She took Donavon. He was a big hit at the nursing home. Everyone loved the little fluff ball. Carol showed him off. Then she began on Tammy. It seems, according to Carol, the DR told her that she was fine and ready to go home. It is interesting the way Carol tries to manipulate conversations and events. It is especially interesting how she tries to work the 'going home' angle. We know that no one there has or will tell Carol that she is okay to go home. She tells us, practically, in every visit, that someone has told her that there is nothing wrong with her, and she can go home. This is not ever the case.

She seems to pick those times that Tammy is alone to try hardest. She knows that I am less affected by her manipulations. I do not have the emotional ties and feelings of guilt that Tammy has. It will remain that most visits will be both of us.

Tuesday, June 15th

Cara called us this morning. Today is Carol's 'Care Plan Meeting'. We meet at the nursing home at Eleven AM. We met Eva Leonard, a nurse practitioner. She is taking care of Carol. We filled her in on Carol's history. We told her some of Carol's past, key influences, work history, and medical history. She was very supportive of our efforts to take care of Carol. She has been working at North Point for eleven years with Alzheimer's patients. It was a productive meeting. We told them about Carol's migraines. We discussed her chest pains. Eva noted all these things. She put in an order for Carol to see the psychiatrist when he came for his monthly visit.

Eva talked about how difficult this is on the families of the patients. The patient does not know how sick they are. They do not see the effect of the disease. We withstand the worst of it. We live with its devastating effects. She suggested that we look into the support group that meets there on the last Thursday of each month.

After the meeting, we went upstairs to visit Carol. We took her into the courtyard and talked for a while. It was pleasant. We will be picking her up on Saturday for our picnic. We are going to try to make a day thing of it. We will pick her up early and keep her until evening. This was a stress free visit. That is a great thing. We stayed until lunchtime. Eva told us that they have Carol help with putting the trays away after meals. Part of their plan is to keep her busy.

Activity is good for her. As long as she stays busy, she does not think so much about her situation. It will also help Carol to feel needed. As bad as Jim was, she felt needed. She <u>had</u> to take care of him. She felt like someone needed her, even if he did not appreciate it. In her ramblings here at the house, she always talked about needing to be helping.

Perhaps that is the appeal of the bad boys; they need to be saved. Now, after years of trying to save Jim Young, it is Carol's time for rescue. Interestingly enough, Jim has called several times asking about Carol and complaining about how quiet it is at home. He does not know where she is living, nor will he know.

We found some new information online. It was through the American Health Assistance Foundation. The website is <u>www. ahaf.com</u>. From there we accessed the Alzheimer's Family Relief Program. That website is <u>http://www.ahaf.com/afrp/afrp.htm</u>. There was information on a variety of programs. Some may work for some while others work for others. The key is to search through every resource you can find. You never know when you will find that one piece of information, or that one program, or that one fund, which will fit your unique situation.

Wednesday, June 16th

This is a far-reaching disease. While chatting with friends online in an open forum chat room, I mentioned about Carol and Alzheimer's disease. It seemed everyone had some experience with it, or had encountered it in some way. There is great therapy in knowing you are not facing something alone. While they are not actually here with us, they have been where we are. Even in the horror stories, and there are many; there is a ray of hope. The key is to cling to the hope, cling to the humor, and lose the rest.

The days are becoming more our own again. There are still small things that need doing, but this is less of our day. Tammy visited Carol later this evening. Tammy is not feeling well today. She said her visit was good. She had problems finding Carol. Carol was on the other wing helping a patient get into bed. She was in the C wing. The staff on the Amelia wing says they have a hard time keeping Carol in their wing. She knows how to operate the doors. A green button has to be pushed to open the doors. It is on a timer. Most of the patients are not fast enough to push the button and get to the door before it relocks. Carol does not walk the fastest in the world, but she apparently walks fast enough to work the doors. They allow her free reign throughout the facility. It is only a problem when she gets near the elevators. They are inoperable when someone with a bracelet is too close to the sensor. She followed Tammy to the elevator tonight and the doors would not shut. Staff escorted her away from the doors so Tammy could leave. She returned home to me sleeping on the couch.

We think we have figured out how to get her to stay there. She should be content to be there once Grammy is there. Tammy has talked to Cara about rooming Carol and Mary together. This would give Carol someone there with which to spend time. It would also give her a responsibility. That would fulfill a couple of Carol's needs and alleviate one of her worries.

Thursday, June 17th

We will try to visit earlier today. Yesterday, Carol told Tammy she was worried all day because we had not been there. We have Ian with us. Carol loves Ian. He will be a big hit at the nursing home. We have to go to mom and dad's house to work on dad's computer. Dad seems to find new and interesting ways to assist his computer in not working. When we leave there, we will go to North Point.

We are back at home now. We decided to reverse our plans. We went to North Point first. Ian was a big hit, of course. All of the staff thought he was the cutest little thing. He likes Carol. She held him for most of the visit.

There was a problem with today's visit. It was not the visit that was a problem, but what we discovered during the visit. Carol saw the doctor yesterday. We found this out today. Carol told us that he said there was nothing wrong with her. We hear this everyday. Tina, the activities coordinator confirmed that Carol did see the doctor and he did tell her that there was nothing wrong with her. This creates a problem in that Carol now thinks she does not need to be in the nursing home. She is back to her 'I have so much to do' speeches. We will have to talk to the doctor and explain the situation to him. He simply cannot tell her there is nothing wrong with her and leave it at that. That will not work with Carol. We diverted her this time by using Grammy.

This is the double-edged sword. The medicine helps Carol's thinking processes. This is a great thing. It is frustrating to her when she cannot think or remember her thoughts. It is frustrating for us to reiterate the same basic facts repeatedly. In this, the Aricept is a good thing. The other side of the sword is in the same thing. Having more clarity makes it harder to convince Carol that she needs to be in the nursing home. She said that a couple times in this visit. Tina misdirected her once by telling her that North Point was so much more than a nursing home. This will not continue to work.

Friday, June 18th

Today is the first day of one very busy weekend. It is just after eight AM. We have Ian for the rest of the weekend. Tammy has not been sleeping well. She has physical therapy today. The picnic is tomorrow. During the summer, we host a picnic for about fifty people every other weekend. The picnic is on Saturday this weekend to avoid having it on Father's Day. We will have Carol most of that day. Then, that evening, my oldest daughter's children will be over to spend the night. We are taking all of them to church with us Sunday morning. Some time Sunday afternoon, they will begin going home. As I said, this will be a busy weekend.

Evening

We finally made it to see Carol around seven-thirty PM. We had Ian with us again. He was the hit of the ward. Carol did not see us come in. She was enjoying her evening snack. We went to the courtyard to talk. She talked about the doctor telling her she was getting out. We let that pass without comment. She asked about Grammy. Tammy told her it would be, at least, the first week in July. I tossed in 'two weeks' before it registered with Carol that she should be out before the first week in July. We talked about the picnic tomorrow and of our plan to pick her up in the morning. She wanted to be sure she had enough time to spruce up a bit. Even though she still has problems, she does seem more concentrated. What she does remember, she remembers well.

We gave her a pad and two pens. She gets frustrated when she thinks of something to ask us and forgets when we are there. This way she can write it down for us. It will help also that we will be able to write down the answers. She can read, rather than try to remember everything we tell her. She liked that idea.

We came home to sad news. A friend from the chat room passed away. He was forty-nine. He recently had by-pass surgery. This evening, he had a heart attack and the hospital was not able to resuscitate him. We will have a special time set aside at the picnic tomorrow to remember him.

Saturday, June 19th

Tammy has reverted to mama sleep. Since Ian is here, she has not been sleeping well. She sleeps so lightly that she is awake more than asleep. We were up early today, but she lay on the couch 'for an hour' with Ian to sleep. She wanted to wake before nine AM to go get Carol. I was going to let her sleep until nine-thirty. She was sleeping so well, I could not bring myself to wake her. When she woke on her own just before then, she began her rushing. It was slow rushing.

She picked up Carol at five after ten. Carol was ready to go. They went to Kroger and got more picnic supplies. Then they came home. While they were gone, I sliced the onions and tomatoes and prepared the condiments cooler. We did not have to leave right away, so we relaxed just a bit. Eventually, we loaded the truck and headed to the park.

Our regular spot was available. We set up and our friends began arriving. The weather was great. It was sunny, but not too hot. It was breezy, which kept the temperature down. Steve did the grill master duties. That freed me up to socialize and get the sympathy card signed by everyone. There were a lot of new faces and first timers there today. It was a great time. Carol enjoyed herself immensely. As Tammy puts it, she had a ball.

When the picnic ended and we came home, Carol was trying to figure out a way to stay here at the house. While there is no problem with her staying here overnight at times, but we feel it is too soon right now. She has to be more indoctrinated to staying at the nursing home at night. She worried about us having to go back out to take her home. She actually used the word 'home' to describe North Point. Somewhere in her head, she realizes that is where she lives.

My oldest grandson, Chris, came around seven-forty-five. Kody and the Kyleigh-bug were in the van, so we took Carol outside to meet them. Carol has now met my four grandkids. She thought they were just beautiful. As an unbiased observer, I have to agree with her assessment. Ian was sleeping, so Tammy took Chris with her to take Carol home.

As Tammy took her home, she referred to it as home even more. We reinforce this by calling it home as well. She talked about how much fun she had at the picnic. Tammy explained to her, that was how it was going to be. She would stay there and we would be picking her up to take her places, like picnics, and yard sales, and other things. Carol decided that that would not be such a bad thing.

Little by little, she is accepting that this is going to be her life. She still has moments where the disease clouds the need for such a life. She is, however, less resistant to the idea now. North Point has not had to call us since the second day about her behavior. They are using our suggestions about keeping her busy. It is a symbiotic relationship. It benefits them both for her to stay busy. I know they do not need her to gather the trays after a meal. They do not need her to fold towels and wash clothes. They do not need her to pass out or gather the bibs at mealtime. They do need her help in her behavior. We appreciate their humanity in they way they treat patients.

Sunday, June 20th

Father's Day

We enjoyed ourselves at church this morning. It was a refresher course. It has been a long time since either of us has been to church with an infant and a five year old. We survived. After church, it was time for children to pick up children. Chris left around one PM with his dad, Ross. Chasity came around two to pick up Ian. She, Heather, and Witter-bug stayed for a little while to visit. When they left, we were simply bathed in the silence of the house. It was sweet music. We decided it was time for a nap.

The nap is over. It is time to go visit Carol.

Carol seemed a bit more addled than usual today. She was talking more nonsensical. She was concerned about staying in the nursing home. We reiterated to her that this was where she slept, ate her meals, and received her meds. She was still able to go out with us as often as we liked. She was still able to go to the picnics and to yard sales with Tammy. We did explain that even though the doctor told her that there was nothing wrong with her, physically, that she still had Alzheimer's disease. She did still need treatment. She told us that she had never seen that on paper. She insists that she still has a paper that tells her she is fine, even though she has yet to produce it.

While we were in the courtyard, two other patients visited our table to talk. Before coming to North Point Carol had never seen them. She tried to convince them that she had heard all about them. Myrtle was a seamstress that sewed rubber during WWII. She was from Cuyahoga Falls, Ohio. The other was the wife of a shoemaker. "He could make a pair of shoes like new." Her name was Ocelia and she was from McKenna, Kentucky. They bore many of the same traits as Carol. It was interesting that Carol recognized that they needed help, but does not see that in her.

We took Carol to her room to show her the pad and pens that we brought a few days ago. She talked as if she had not seen them. They were on her bed on top of clothes she had folded. She had no idea where she had put the pens. They may be in her purse. We did not go there. We left after an hour.

Monday, June 21st

It was a slow Monday. Tammy did the physical torture thing. After lunch, we drove to Frankfort where I put in an application with the state. We took our time driving down and back, enjoying the time out and alone. We stopped and ordered the flowers for the visitation and funeral of Jody. We will pick them up tomorrow on the way to Frankfort.

We were tired from the weekend, so, we decided not to go to the nursing home tonight. Tammy called to have them tell Carol that we were okay, and not to worry. She went out for a few minutes while I cooked supper. Later this evening we went to see my daughter and to return the stroller. She could not get it in her car when she picked up Ian on Sunday.

It is just after eight o'clock and it feels like it should be midnight. I can see now how much better it is to have Carol in a nursing home here in Lexington. There are times, and will be times, that it is very difficult to squeeze everything into the day and still have time to visit Carol. If she were in Nicholasville, it would be even more difficult. North Point is still riding the edge of 'too good to be true'. Everyone we meet that is associated with them impresses us. I am sure there might be a disgruntled employee somewhere. We just have not met them yet. No one is perfect. There is no perfect nursing home. This one, however, is far and above others, we looked into. This is not to say that others are not as good, just not as good a fit for us. We are happy with the choice we made.

Tuesday, June 22nd

I had a job test to take this morning. Tammy visited Carol while I was testing. When we got back to the same place, she told me about her visit. Carol started the 'getting out of here' speech. She told Tammy, "You are not going to like this, but it is just the way it is going to be. I am going home." Tammy told her, "You are not going to like this, but no you are not". Tammy then began to tell her all the reasons that she would not be going back to Jim Young or Florida. She pointed out to Carol that she was not capable of taking care of herself. She restated to Carol that she does have Alzheimer's disease.

She told Carol about her conversation with Jim. Jim called and talked as if he was going to come get Carol and take her back because he could not pay his bills. Carol could not believe Jim would say that. Every visit, we are going to state this fact. Carol has Alzheimer's disease.

All in all, Tammy said it was a decent visit. It did Tammy well. This is still very difficult for her, and may always be that way. Carol's condition will deteriorate. Spending time with her will get more difficult. The worse her condition gets, the less she will be argumentative about it. Seeing her will get harder and easier at the same time. That is the paradox of Alzheimer's disease. In the final stages, the patient is very docile. It will be more difficult to see her like that, but at the same time, will be easier to see her less quarrelsome.

We are still plugging the Grammy aspect. Carol will have to be there to care for Grammy.

Wednesday, June 23rd

This morning was Jody's funeral. That was difficult. There were many strained emotions amongst the family. Tammy and I are both somewhat sensitive to strong emotions. Tammy says it is not a good day to be empathic.

We stayed busy most of the morning and early afternoon, so we went to see Carol this evening. She was just finishing her supper when we got there. They had her in the stockings to reduce swelling. We talked to the nurse while Carol finished eating. They had noticed the swelling and put them on her. Carol intimated that she had seen the doctor, but this was not the case. The floor nurse also told us that Carol had used a bent up clothes hanger to get the bio out of the case by her door. She claimed that it showed how much money someone owed her. She has hidden it away somewhere.

We took Carol outside to chat. She began almost immediately on complaining about being in the nursing home. They do not allow her to come outside enough. They do not let her stay up late. We already know that these things are not true. She tries to play the guilt card when she can. We explained to her why she has to be in the nursing home. We I told her it was because she was sick, she did not like it. She knows she is sick, but does not want to face up to it. As if not accepting it in her head will make it go away. She tries to evade the fact that she has Alzheimer's disease.

At one point, she asked why she had to have it. She asked the question as if she thought that she might have had a choice. Tammy explained that it was genetic. There is a gene in her family that carries this disease. Carol's dad had it. Carol's mom has it. Carol has it. While she was explaining this, it occurred to me that this was her fear. Tammy is very intelligent. She learns at a voracious level. Her thirst and hunger for knowledge is enormous. She looks at her mom and remembers the woman she was. She is scared that the person her mom has become is her fate. This terrifies her. She was right. This is not a good day to be empathic.

Carol cried and begged us to take her out of here. I explained to her that she was sick. This is the only way we have to take care of her. This is the first time in years that Tammy has lain down at night and not worried about Carol's well-being. She does not have to worry that the house is going to burn because Carol forgot to turn of the stove. She does not have to worry that Carol is on the road somewhere. She does not have to worry that she has invited some harmful stranger into the house, convinced that she has known him for years. North

Point gives Tammy peace of mind in some areas. Some other areas will never know peace over this.

Depending on weather and physical therapy, we may pick Carol up on Friday morning. Tammy wants to do the yard sale and get it done. She asked Carol if she wanted to help. Carol answered nonchalantly, "If that is what you want". Just moments earlier, she was lamenting that she could not get out. She was bemoaning her fate. When, a seeming answer comes, she is subdued.

During the visit, I returned my brothers call. He was not home, but I did speak with Donna. It turns out that this is the nursing home where her granny lived. Her aunt still brings dogs here to visit with the residents. I think that is a much better word than 'patients' is. Resident says what it is. This is where Carol is going to live. As much as she dislikes the idea, this is where she is safe and cared for. This is where she will remain. She is beginning to understand that. I think that is the reason she fights so much harder these past few days. Regardless, our resolve is strong. She is home.

Still, it tears Tammy's heart out that she cannot care for her mom. Tammy has done it since she was around twelve. For years, she has covered up for her mom's forgetfulness. She has paid her bills for her. She did her banking when Carol would forget how to add or subtract. She has helped her run her business. Carol gets upset when she cannot remember things. She would transfer this anger to customers. Tammy smoothed many customers. Taking care of Carol has just been part of Tammy's life for many years. It was just part of her life. It seemed natural for her to do so.

Thursday, June 24th

Carol will be tickled. We have Ian today. We are going to try to visit early. We want to be known for showing up at different times. This is not because we suspect the nursing home of any impropriety. We want to meet as much of the staff caring for Carol as possible. We also want to alleviate any worries that Carol might have if we are not there early. In addition, this frees our afternoons up for other things. Visiting Carol is part of our daily routine, but if we put it off too late, it can become a chore. It is essential that not happen. We do not want to look at visiting her begrudgingly. While it is often not a pleasurable event, it does not need to become a task.

We are back from North Point. Carol's social worker told us the Carol was upset this morning. She insisted that her husband was coming to get her. She thinks because she does not know some of the people that they know nothing about her. Therefore, she tries her bluffs. They do not work. They gave her meds to calm her. Tammy told the social worker to expect paper work from the Division of Mental Health regarding Carol.

Tammy noticed that Carol's gold chain necklace was missing. When questioned about it, Carol told her that it was at home. The social worker suggested that we take it home if we found it. While Tammy kept Carol busy, I went to her room to look for it. I hung her clothes in the closet. She had them hanging on the bulletin board and on the wicker heart over her bed. I found her purse under her clothes. I found the necklace in it.

I also found several scraps of paper throughout her purse where she had written notes to Jim. Most were imploring him to come get her because these people were driving her crazy. One, however, told him to stay away from this state. I even found an extra pair of glasses. There is no telling from where they came. I gathered the errant scraps of paper, put them in my pocket, and replaced her purse.

I joined Tammy, Carol, and Ian in the courtyard. There was a nice breeze and we enjoyed the conversation until Ian began to get fussy. We told Carol that we would be there to get her tomorrow if all went well. If we were not able to get her tomorrow, we would get her Saturday. We got home shortly after noon. We still have much more running to do.

Once home, we called Laura at the Division of Mental Health to give her North Point's address. We have to have the paper work in at least ten days before the hearing on the twelfth of July. This should give us plenty of time.

Friday, June 25th

I went early to get Carol. Before I signed her out, Eva, the nurse practitioner, asked me to talk. It seems that Carol has head lice. They had ordered shampoo for her and needed her to stay for treatment. She thought that Carol might have picked it up at the picnic. I think it is more likely that she picked it up there at the nursing home. It was a moot point. She has it. It needs to be treated. Therefore, I left Carol there for the day. She did not even see me, so she did not know what she was missing.

Carol was going to help Tammy with a yard sale. Tammy did not need her help, but thought it would be a good outdoor excursion for Carol. Three hours into the sale, the thunder and lightning ended it.

Saturday, June 26th

I picked Carol up this morning at eight-forty five. I brought most of the yard sale items outside before I left. Tammy put out the clothes and arranged thing while I was picking up Carol. When I told Carol I was taking her home, she perked right up. I reiterated that I was taking her to 'my' home for the day. She told me that she needed to get out of the nursing home. She had it on good authority that Jim was getting worse. "He may be a jackass," she said, "but he is my jackass". I assured her the Jim was just fine, or at least he was, when he called earlier in the week to tell us he missed her money. That stopped all conversation about Jim Young.

While driving home, we talked about Tammy going to Florida in July to get the kids and to put plans of moving Grammy into motion. I told Carol the Tammy was going to get a notarized letter from her brother Fred. This is so Tammy could make decisions concerning Mary. Carol remembered that Fred was living in Jessamine Co. She mentioned the paper that TJ took out of the holder by her door. If you recall, the nursing home staff told us that Carol had used a bent hanger to remove that paper. Even in casual conversation, she is very careful not to accept any blame for anything.

Once here, she wasted no time getting on Tammy's nerves. She began folding and unfolding clothes on the tables. She was moving items around the tables. She took clothes off the hangers and put them over a bar stool. Tammy re-hung all the clothes. She kept putting purses on top of the clothes. Tammy kept putting them back. She was freezing. Then she was hot. She had two tops on and one of my sweaters at first. Then she took off the sweater. Then she came out of the bathroom in her bra. She had taken off both tops and was putting one back on.

She talked nonstop to customers. She talked nonstop to anyone in earshot. She was inside. Then she was outside. She was not satisfied to be in any place for more than a few minutes. About an hour before Tammy was going to start breaking down and bringing things in, she asked me is she could do that. I told her that she could, in an hour, when Tammy was ready. She went immediately outside and began trying to pack it in. Tammy stopped her and asked what she was doing. She told her she was taking things in. Tammy told her she was not ready to do that. She changed her story. "I am just moving this one dress," she said.

When we took her home, she was happy to be back. It is odd that while she is there, she is constantly talking about not wanting to be there. Now, she is happy to be back there.

I have figured out this much; when she talks about 'them' driving her crazy there, she is not talking about the staff. She is talking about the other patients. Physically, she is probably one of the top patients. Her neurosis is less demonstrative than most as well. Therefore, she is an easier patient with which to work. Add to this that she helps with the other patients and she stays busy. The staff allows her to 'help'. She thinks her role is much more vital than it really is, but that works for all. Getting Grammy here is going to help a lot.

She needs to be needed. She has to feel like she has a reason to be around. The nursing home is doing that as best they can. She has great difficulty being the one taken care of. She will, very begrudgingly, allow you to help her. This part of the transition from independence to dependence has been the hardest for Carol. She fights it, but does not even know what she is fighting. When she would run back to Jim in the past, she probably did not know what she was wanting; only that it was met in him. That need is not being met now. At least, it is not being met completely.

Sunday, June 27th

We did not visit Carol today. Our own life intruded. Tammy was to perm my sister's hair around two pm. We were out in the morning. We went to the grocery in the late morning to early afternoon. Then Tammy went in search of a perm for Kathy. Kathy did not get here until four. Tammy permed her hair while I cooked supper. Kathy and Bobby stayed to eat and visit a little while. By the time they left, it was too late to go for a visit. I am sure that Carol will not remember that she did not visit, but Tammy will.

That is part of the difficulty with this ordeal. It is part of your life, yet it is something else as well. It is an addition. You still have to do all the things that filled your days and nights before this happened. Moreover, you have to squeeze another hour or so out of each day. That hour is not enough and too much all at the same time. Until you are here, you will never fully understand that. You want to spend more time but you cannot. You just do not have that much time. Then, more time is difficult in as much as being with her reminds you of how far removed she has become from the person you knew. There are personality traits that you recognize that are interwoven with the disease. Tammy says that Carol is like a puzzle with all the pieces in the wrong places. All of her is still there. Her meanness, stubbornness, humor, and intelligence are all still there. It is as if she has gone through a transporter and put back together incorrectly. Her reactions are all wrong. In time, we will come to know that Carol as well as the old Carol. Then the disease will progress and she will be different again. There will be missing pieces of the puzzle then.

Alcoholism affects the entire family of the alcoholic. The affect is proportionate to the closeness of the relationship to the alcoholic. Alcoholism is a disease with hope, though. The alcoholic can stay away from the cause of his/her sickness and lead a normal life. Families can heal. Yes, that is a gross simplification of a complex process.

Alzheimer's disease affects the entire family of the patient. The affect is proportionate to the closeness of the relationship to the patient. Currently, Alzheimer's is a disease without hope. One cannot impede the progression of this disease. You cannot turn off that part of the brain. There are no meetings where you learn to control your Alzheimer's disease. It is a degenerative disease of the brain. Its affects will affect you the rest of your life.

Carol is not going to get better. Figuratively, she is not coming back home. As I spoke to her last week about the need to be in a nursing facility, this is the best way we know how to care for her right now.

There is not enough hugging in my arms to hug this away. It hurts me that it hurts her. She tries not to let me see how much it is hurting her, so that I do not hurt too. It does not work. Tammy says that I make it bearable. She will deal with it the best that she can. Some nights, it is overwhelming. Sometimes, only tears will dilute the pain. Tammy says there are times you hold back the tears for fear that you will drown in them. She is afraid if they start, they will not stop. Welcome to Alzheimer's disease.

Monday, June 28th

I had a few appointments this morning that would take me into early afternoon. Tammy went to visit Carol while I was taking care of my business. I prefer that I go with her, since Carol seems to try the whole guilt trip when I am not there. While inside one of my appointments, I left my cell phone in the truck. When I returned to it, I had a missed call from Tammy. I called to find her upset. Carol tried the guilt trip. She used the 'how would you feel if it were you' and 'I am just going to sit here and cry my eyes out'.

Tammy told her that we were not going to do the whole guilt trip thing today. One of the nurses thought that was hilarious. There are several problems. Carol does not want them to check her hair everyday. She thinks when they say that, that they are talking about a getting her hair done. They seem to be somewhat unprepared for head lice. They have restricted her movements. She is not allowed off the ward. This means she cannot go outside. That does not sit well with Carol.

Eva, the nurse practitioner, told Tammy that they would prefer that she stay at the facility. Tammy told them that she would take her mother anywhere she wished. She also told them she was taking Carol to the picnic on Saturday. Eva said that she would prefer if we did not. Tammy repeated that she was going to take Carol to the picnic. There was nothing else said about it.

This is a cooperative effort in the treatment of Carol. We have not, nor will we, give any facility, carte blanche, in Carol's treatment. We will remain the ultimate authority in this. We will heed medical advice. We will consider medical opinions. We will not, however, lock her in a ward and walk away. We are entrusting North Point as our partner in this venture. They are our surrogates in our absence. We are not involved in the daily planning of meals. We are not working in the laundry. We are not medical professionals. We are her loved ones. We are her family. If we felt her treatment was not right, we would move her. When you get right down to the bottom line, they work for us. This is not a power trip. This is not an ego trip. It is just the facts.

When you send your child to school, you are entrusting the school with the education and welfare of your child. You remain the parent. You decide if Johnny is going to participate in track and field or not. You are the best prepared to make those decisions. It is a joint venture. You accept certain professional recommendations. Ultimately, you will make the decisions. This is a similar scenario.

We got a new dog today. A while back, we had no pets. The cat was AWOL. We had talked to a friend about a boxer. We had talked to another friend about a miniature Pomeranian. A month ago, the boxer's owners told us they had decided to keep him. As you know, Tammy had her heart set on the Pomeranian and got him.

Sunday evening, Tammy heard a cat mewing outside and went to investigate. There was the Dude. He was ready to come home. He strolled in as if he owned the place. He jumped up on the waterbed and rolled over. His whirlwind vacation tour of the neighborhood was over. He was home. He and Donavon mostly ignore each other. Although they are different species, they are about the same size, so it worked.

This afternoon, Brandy called me to tell me the boxer owners needed to place him. They were moving and could not take him. We relayed the message to bring him on over. They brought him around 9PM. His name is Malcolm. Malcolm is approximately eighty pounds. Donavon is about eight pounds and Dude is around ten to twelve pounds. Malcolm is a big, dumb, lovable, idiot. Donavon is temporarily scared of him. Dude is wary of him. Malcolm is intrigued by both but scared of the one that hisses at him.

It seems like taking in the unwanted is one of our weaknesses. Do not call me if you have a pet you cannot keep. We are slightly over our limit now.

Tuesday, June 29th

Tammy and I were in separate vehicles this morning when I had to be close to North Point. I called and she was on her way there. We decided to meet there. I was about five minutes closer.

I took Carol to the courtyard area to chat, as is our custom. When we settled out there, she told me she was not allowed out there. According to her, she was to be inside for nine days. This was something to do with the head lice treatment. I waited for Tammy so we could address it with her together. Tammy arrived and we shared the news. While Carol and Tammy talked, I went inside to find the real story. The nurse on duty told me that Carol was restricted in going out into the courtyard because she would follow other patients into other wards. They wanted to keep the problem as contained as possible. The nurse I spoke with hated that for her. Carol loves being outside.

Carol is allowed to be outside when supervised. She can go there with us anytime. I informed the nurse that we would be taking Carol to the picnic on Saturday. I told her that we had informed Eva of this decision. Eva issued the orders to keep her contained. The nurse said that Carol had to be retreated within seven to ten days. Her original treatment was on Friday, June 25th. Seven days would be Friday, July 1st. She can be retreated the day before the picnic. This would free her for release on that Saturday. If this is to be the first 'push' issue, then, so be it.

Part of the deal with Carol being in this place was the capability for her to be outside at times. This will remain in effect. I can understand if she has pneumonia or some sickness that would make it detrimental to be outside of the ward. Lice do not leap from head to head. There has to be a shared comb, or slinging hair. Carol's hair is too short to sling. This unit's paranoia will not be placated at the expense of locking Carol in the ward. Nuff said !

Today, we began telling Carol about the trip to Florida to gather the children. I will be working in Louisville. Tammy will be in Florida for at least four days. There will not be a visit from us during that time. We want her prepared. She will forget. We will remind her. She will forget. We will remind her.

We met part of Mrs. Macy's family today. Her son was in from North Dakota for a visit. Her daughter lives in Lexington. Mrs. Macy and Carol are practically inseparable. They were happy to meet us. We talked to her daughter for a few minutes about the disease. At one point, she had her father at North Point as well.

Wednesday, June 30

We took Malcolm and Ian on today's visit to Carol. She had a boxer before Tammy was born. Her name was Baby. Tammy says she heard all about it. Carol held Ian and talked about Malcolm and Baby. We reminded her about the trip coming up. We reminded her that Tammy was going to be away for a few days so she would not worry. I told Carol that I would be only an hour away in case of an emergency. Ian and Malcolm were big hits. The staff loves when we visit. We bring the most interesting things.

Carol took a tumble this morning at the nursing home. She was walking and decided to change direction. The direction she intended was not the floor but that is where she ended. She was okay, but a little stiff. She will most likely be bruised tomorrow.

Our visits and Carols being there is becoming more routine every day. Being at North Point (and complaining about it) is just what is. This is a good thing. Less stress is good for everyone involved. A less stressed Carol is much more pleasant. She is still going to complain. She is still going to find things that she does not like. That is fine. That is just personality coming out in her. It is good to see things the disease has not yet robbed.

A less stressed Carol produces a less stressed Tammy. This is a very good thing. The stress-filled visits take a lot out of her. Many times after a visit, she will have a headache or come home and lay down. I hate what this has done to all of us.

Carol does not like Eva. She refuses to remember her name. I think that is a healthy bit of defiance. Carol identifies her only as the woman in the white coat. The dislike stems from Eva's zealous method in treating Carol. She went a little overboard in the lice treatment. She restricted her time outside the ward. This made her Carol's enemy. We told her that she did not have to like Eva. It was not required. We explained that Eva was a competent nurse and was there to help Carol, but Carol does not have to like her. They will not be going to the Spring dance together.

Thursday, July 1st

I was in Louisville a good part of the day. Tammy had Ian for the day. Tammy's visit was good. The nursing home still has some problems about Carol's head lice. They seem to not understand it. I do not know how often they encounter it, but they seem ill equipped for it.

Friday July 2nd

We took Ian and Heather for today's visit. We requested to talk to the head of nursing. They had called and told us they refused to allow Carol to leave with us for the picnic. They went as far as to say that they would discharge her if we took her out. This was during a phone call. It needed to be discussed in person.

We talked with the head of nursing. She felt that it would be detrimental to Carol's treatment to be offsite. We could not understand this. She was not going to be involved in any activity that might make the problem worse. She would be sitting at a picnic table talking and eating. They decided they would call the doctor and see what he recommended. The regular doctor was out of town. The nursing home director was out of town. We stated our case with the nursing director and the ombudsman.

We went outside to visit with Carol. She took her lunch outside with us. While we were outside, Eva came to tell us that they had reached a decision. When Tammy returned, she told me that we had won. We would be allowed to take Carol to the picnic. The ombudsman agreed with us that she could not see any harm in an outside visit.

It was a small victory. You have to take those where you can get them. If you roll over and play dead; they will always expect you to do that. No matter how good a facility is, there will always be those that will take the easy way, if you allow it. If they expect you to question decisions, they will make sure of their answers before you ask.

Saturday, July 3rd

Inclement weather has caused cancellation of the picnic. We still picked Carol up and brought her to the house. Tammy leaves for Florida this evening and wants to spend time with her mom before she goes. We grilled out burgers and dogs on the gas grill under the roof of the porch. There was slight intermittent rain. A friend and his son came by and had lunch with us. It was a good time.

After lunch and before taking her home, Tammy checked Carol's head for lice and nits. She found no live bugs and just a few nits, which she removed. This was part of our concession to the nursing home. It seems they have been treating Carol with lice shampoo every two days. This is creating sores in Carol's head. Again, I must say, they seem to be stupefied by this process. It is simple. You treat, check, remove, and then retreat in seven to ten days. Continual treating is not removing the nits. Therefore, you are not solving the problem. We hope that checking and removing them here will fix this. Time will tell.

Monday, July 19th

Carol waivers between calling North Point home and telling us that she "has GOT to go." The emphasis is on the 'got' to insure you understand that it is a needful thing. She goes back and forth, sometimes in the same conversation. There are 'things' which require her immediate attention.

She worries about us and then forgets us. She tells me that she worries that I am working too much, which, of course, I am. She still fails to see the inconsistencies. It is as if she forgets what she says as soon as she says it. Talking to her is like a rambling diatribe. No statement is predicated on the last statement, nor has any reference to the next statement. The proper response to must of the things she says, is "OK". Some things we address if they have an immediate impact. Most things, however, are inconsequential. That, in itself, is a sad fact. Time and this disease have reduced her to where someone else makes the major decisions in her life. Fortunately, it is someone that cares about her now.

Sunday, August 1st

It has been weeks since I had opportunity to sit and write. I have been putting in ten, twelve, and fourteen-hour days. That is over for now. Life is returning to what we hesitantly call normal. I am not quite sure we have any 'normal' days, but then, that would be the opposite of normal for us.

To catch up: Sierra has quit one Sonic and has been hired at another. Chris is still looking for work. Chelsea is still Chelsea. Kyle is still being an eight year old on summer break. Last, but not least, Carol is still about the same. What delusions she has, have become routine. Every now and then, she throws a new curve in, but they are generally manageable.

Her latest wrinkles include telling us that she sees Jim driving up and down the road in front of the nursing home every day. It seems that, according to her sources, he has bought a piece of ground up the road and is conducting some sort of business there. In reality, Jim is still in Florida.

In one recent visit, Carol was looking for something in her purse. She pulled out her pen and it was covered with something yellow. I knew immediately what it was. Carol has a thing about putting the condiments she does not use with her meal in her purse. We are not quite sure why that is. It is just something that she does now. Well, this was her butter. It was melted and everywhere. She blamed the staff there for putting it in her purse, of course. She used her pepper pack to scrap the butter off her glass case. And the conversation goes on.

She seems to be in a clothing swap program. She is often wearing someone else's clothes when we visit. Last week, we suspect it was Mrs. Macy's clothes. When we visited her room, looking for her, during one visit, all her clothes were hanging on things in the room. They were everywhere except the closet. We put her clothes in the closet. We told her this when we did find her so she would not think someone had stolen them. While going through her clothes to see what she still had left, we found one of Chelsea's bras and one of Sierra's tops. Apparently, she 'jacked' them during her visit to the house. She is certainly sneaky.

She does have a new trick. She manipulates the staff at the nursing home into calling us several times a week. Sometimes it is a daily thing. She tells them that she has not seen us for days and she is so worried about us. They feel sorry for her and call us. Usually, we have seen her the day before.

We took her to the bi-weekly picnic we hold last weekend. The picnic is held on Sunday afternoon. She called us on the Saturday before, crying, because she was afraid she had missed the picnic. Well, she did not call, one of the nurses called for her. I assured her she had not missed the picnic, it was the next day. She calmed down and was fine.

Sunday morning, the phone rings. It is Carol. She is afraid she has missed the picnic again. Tammy talked to her and assured her that she had not and that she was leaving in minutes to come pick her up. One hour later, when Tammy arrives at the nurses station on Carol's ward, Carol is crying to the nurses that she has not heard from us in days and needs to call us. Tammy assures me that this is not Alzheimer's disease working. This is just Carol manipulating people as she often does.

The hearing on guardianship has been moved to a later date. Carol's court appointed attorney has been in contact with us and is going to recommend that we be granted full guardianship. We have also been in contact with the social worker in charge of the case. He, too, is going to recommend that Tammy be made full guardian.

More and more, this has become part of our routine. It is just a part of what we do. We do not visit at a set time. We do not visit every day. I think this is important to both Tammy and Carol. It gives Tammy a breather and it lets Carol begin to make a life in the nursing home. Carol talks less about getting out. She still has her crying jags, where she is miserable and better off dead, but they are getting less and farther between. This is becoming the norm. Order is encroaching on the chaos. The nurses and staff have been informed not to call us every time Carol cries. They are to assure her that everything is all right and to remind her that we were just there.

We are still working on the Mary Oliver situation, but even this does not seem to concern Carol as it did before. She is adapting to the change, as are all of us.

The kids take turns about going to visit with Carol. It is harder for them to see her there. This way we do not overburden Carol and the kids have more time to adjust to the situation. Chris was not here during the ordeal. He has the hardest time visiting her. Kyle, Chella, and Sierra were here for the home time with Carol. They readily accept that this is the best-case scenario for the situation as it was. It still breaks Tammy's heart that her mom is in a nursing home. I think it always will. Her mind knows that this is the only solution. Her heart knows this as well, but is far less accepting of the logic of it. This is a wound that time will never heal.

This is the close of the Carol Ordeal. It has ventured from the fields of an ordeal to the plains of the routine. It absorbs less and less of each day. There are still loose ends to tie up. There are still intermittent trips to the fields, but they are fleeting. This is down to the occasional blurb here and there.

I think we are almost ready for the next crisis.

Tammy's turn at the keyboard

When all of this began, I told myself "I can do this." I am still trying to convince myself that I can. One of the hardest parts of this for me has been other people that know what we are going through saying "wow, you must have extraordinary strength, stamina, faith, hope, ect." That is not the case at all. Ron and I are ordinary people. Well he is far from ordinary, but my point is there is nothing special about what we are going through. There is nothing special about us. We are just doing what needs to be done to make sure that someone that needs care gets it. The fact that it is my mother makes it personal and more difficult for me but it would not be any different in trying to help a friend going through this.

Last week, even though I knew that Jim was bringing mom to KY, I started having the bad dreams. Not ones related to her, per say, but bad in general. Then came the sense of dread. As the week progressed, the dread got worse. Point of interest here is that I was not dreading caring for my mother but just being with her for long periods of time. My mom has always been my greatest source of strength as well as my greatest fears. She has never been your ordinary soccer mom.

Saturday night, my fears were realized when she spent most of the night and into the wee hours of the morning cussing Jim and wanting to go home. Sunday (Mother's Day) was not much better. I knew that I was going to have to get some professional help somewhere. Therefore, we just dealt with her the best we could and pacified her in any way that we could. Ron got her to agree to go to the doctor for a checkup and if it were ok with the doctor, that he would put her on a bus. We both knew that no doctor would release my mother to go home. That is something that is hard for me to grasp, that she really is the way she is now and we have to tell her little lies to get by.

Monday started out badly and got worse as the day progressed. I finally got her to the hospital and got the medical ball rolling. This whole experience feels like I am on the outside looking in at people I do not really know. It feels surreal to me. I think I am removing myself for the time being to allow me to do what I need to do without thinking about how much this is hurting me. After several hours in the emergency room and several phone calls, it was decided that getting mom into Eastern State Mental Hospital would be the fastest and best way to get her evaluated for the guardianship hearing and to get her some interim medical and psychological care. Needing the sheriff come out and pick her up was like a knife in my heart. I hate this situation, I am so angry. I am upset with Jim for not being a man and taking care of her better , but then again, he never did take care of her or of me and my brother. I am angry at the system for making it so difficult to care for someone with my mom's condition. I am angry at the unfairness of all of this to Ron, my kids and yeah, as selfish as it sounds, to me as well. Finally, I am angry that mom is this way. I know she couldn't prevent the Alzheimer's but I firmly believe if she had not allowed herself to be abused for so many years by Jim that she wouldn't be as confused as she is. I believe in my heart that he broke my mother as much if not more than the disease itself.

By the end of the week, I was exhausted but at least mom was getting the medical attention that she needs and I have accomplished much in the way of contacting nursing homes and getting her SS check safely out of the reach of Jim. That is not to mention how much I have learned about the system and Alzheimer's disease overall. I love to learn, but I would much prefer time to absorb what I have learned rather than having it thrust upon me. However, sometimes you get the information the best way you can and assimilate it later.

We are a couple weeks into this now and emotionally this whole situation is trying to take its toll. It is a trying time. I try to get this done, I try to get that done, and it seems that everyone that is in place to assist people in this type of situation tries to put up roadblocks.

We finally have mom home with us after much fighting with just about everyone in Eastern State. For some reason, Dr. Hawthorne decided that he was going to commit mom to a 60-day involuntary hold. We neither were told about this decision until we got to the guardianship hearing, nor is this what we want. It is a bit ironic that I had to fight to get her in there for the evaluation and then had to battle to get her out of that horrible place.

Let me back up here a minute describe it. The first ward that they had mom on was mostly younger people. It was clean but not necessarily a safe place for her due to the fact that many of the patients there were prone to fight. Mom did well while she was there though, and did not have any major problems. The staff on that ward was courteous, friendly, and seemed to care about what they were doing there. Then they moved mom to the geriatric ward. That place can only be described as hell. It is reminiscent of the old mental institutions of the 1950's where they would take people with mental illness or physical handicaps and then promptly forget them. This place is dirty, reeking of urine, and overall the most dismal place I have ever seen.

The patients are condescended to at best. Most of the time they are simply ignored. No on seems to think that this is a problem. I have seen several male patients with urine on the front of their pants and no one of staff even suggesting that the patient change or shower. Most of them are too busy giggling with each other or reading books or magazines to really have any idea of what is going on in the ward. I heard one staff member tell an obviously severely handicapped woman that since she did not eat at mealtime, she would have to go hungry until morning. This was about 6 pm on Saturday.

Getting my mother out of that place became my obsession. I could not think about anything for very long without trying to come up with a plan. It was always in my head almost like a mantra saying over and over, "I have got to get mom out of there." I was only sleeping in fits and starts. I felt totally wrung out all of the time. If Ron had not been my strength, my rock and my hope, I do not think I could have made it through the last week or so. He is my inspiration to go on. He does not realize that his sweet, gentle strength gives me all I need to continue with this battle.

That brings me to something that I have been thinking a lot about. This situation has been devastating to me. It has changed many of the ways that I used to think. It has been confusing and a bit distracting for the kids. For Ron I know it must be hard to deal with. He has to deal with his own feelings in all of this, and he has to hold me together through my pain and emotional breakdowns. I try so hard not to show him all the pain that I feel. I do not want him to worry about me. I do not want to burden him with my worry, my grief, my sorrow, and my anger. He always seems to know what I am feeling. I guess I am not that good of an actress after all. When all of this is done, I know that he and I will be strengthened by all that we have gone through and our determination to make it right together. We have had a bond almost from the very beginning of our relationship. I don't know how to describe it, but it has always felt to me like Ron and I know each other on such a deep level that we are both a part of the same organism. Yet, we are very individual people over all.

Tuesday June 8,

We have finally gotten mom into a nursing home. North Point has decided that they will take her. Therefore, we packed all of her clothes and took her over there. She is not happy about this. In fact, my mother is rarely happy about anything. I understand that the disease is partially to blame for this but she was never really a happy person to begin with.

Wednesday, the nursing home called and told me that mom was throwing a fit and telling them that her "husband" was coming to get her and that she was not going to stay. Ron and I went over to North Point and took her outside for a little talk. I had a bit of a breakthrough and breakdown combination. There were many things my parents did to me as a child that I cannot get closure on now. She does not remember and he denies that it happened. So for me, talking to her about the past only serves to hurt me more. I want to say at times that she is in a nursing home let them take care of her. That is not a part of who I am. I could never abandon her there. I know how horrible that sounds to most people. The thought of abandoning an old helpless woman to the mercies of a care facility sounds cruel. These are just the things that go through my mind. I want to forget the past. I want to maintain the dignity, strength, and happiness that I have had to struggle so hard to gain. I want to forget that I was ever the child they raised. I do not want to remember that they are my parents. I do not want to know that someday I could be just like them. I know how that sounds. This is one of those 'guess you had to be there' things.

August 19th

Wow, it has been a while since I have written anything. We have had so much going on that I just have not had the time to write. O.K. so that is not technically the only reason. I have to go back in time to write this. I have to feel old hurts, new hurts, and think of the hurts yet to come. If I could distance myself from this and pretend that this is a fiction, I would write every day.

Let me catch my breath and try to make some sense out of the last couple of months. I have stopped going to North Point every day. I know it sounds awful that I do not visit my own mother every day anymore, but honestly, I think this is better for her and for me. When I do go, which is still at least two or three times a week, she seems to be adjusting so much better. Fewer visits end in my frustration at my mom's manipulations. That is one of the hardest parts of all of this. I knew her when she was my mom. I knew her when she still had all of her faculties. Some of what she does now has absolutely nothing to do with having Alzheimer's it is just being Carol Young. The difficulty lies in trying to figure out what is the disease and what is mom.

In July, I went to get the kids from their dad's in FL. I drove down by myself. My car has always been my private place to think. Thirteen hours of thinking is not a good thing for me. I had too much time on my mind. There is so much that I have not been able to allow myself to remember. It is all there somewhere in my head and heart. There were times of great happiness that I do recall and times of great sadness and heartbreak that I cannot bear to remember. While I was heading down there I thought about all the things and all the times that my mom had been there for me and I realized that in writing this I haven't shared many good memories of my mother. There were times in my childhood that I would think my mom was the greatest woman alive. She worked all the time, but if I needed a slumber party, she would put everything aside and throw one. She would take all seventeen of my friends and me skating at the drop of a hat. She would even pay for the ones that did not have money. She would take me shopping when she had extra money and buy me the things that I liked, her tastes and mine varied greatly. I saw her endure beatings from Jim, put on makeup, and go to work with her head held high, trying to maintain her dignity, and at the same time trying to protect me from knowing what a hell her life must have been.

When I was sixteen, I got married. Mom did not want me to marry Ronnie. She did not want me to get married that young. There was no stopping me. I was going to marry this man. She knew how much I loved him. She knew I was just as stubborn as she was. She bought my dress and helped me plan a beautiful wedding even though her heart was breaking. I was the only thing she ever had that she poured her heart into. When my marriage ended, eighteen years later, she was already in the latter part of stage one Alzheimer's but, she never said I told you so. She never judged me for leaving him and finding someone else to love. When I married Ron last year, the disease had progressed rapidly, but mom was still herself enough to tell me if Ron made me happy, then I had her blessing even though she had never met him. They had talked on the phone several times and she told me from the way he spoke of me and us that I was marrying a good man. Mom was right.

When I got back from FL, having all the kids home was almost like a holiday for me. I had missed them to the point of being physically ill. Having them back and all the chaos that comes with three teenagers and an eight year old made me feel like me again. Things like taking Chris and Jordan job hunting, arguing with Sierra about everything Sierra will argue about, planning the school year with Chelsea and Kyle, make me who I am. Those things made me feel like life was almost back to normal. There were still the nagging thoughts in my head that all my business was leading me to neglect mom. I took the kids to see her several times a week when I would go visit. That part was really hard for Chris, he has always been close to her, he was her first grandson, and the only one of her grandchildren that she could be with on a daily basis until Sierra came along. Seeing mom the way she is now is almost too much for him at times. He hates seeing her there. I think part of it is that he is smart enough to know that someday he may need to care for me and for all of our disagreements he couldn't bear the thought of putting me in a nursing home anymore than I can bear the thought of leaving mom there every time I visit. I want my children to know if I am ever the way mom is, that I do not want to be a burden to them I want them to find a place for me and to live their own lives.

July passed chaotically and in several ways slowly. Things returning to almost normal seemed to slow down my brain a bit.

August did not start out good. The kids are like me. They have hordes of friends. I tend to adopt the ones they bring home. I call them my orphans. Most of them have no parents to speak of and love the feeling of belonging to a family. I love kids and cannot bear to think that there are children that are unloved or unwanted at home so I tend to take them in. One of my orphans was Tommy.

On to the next crisis. On August 4th, Ron and I had gone grocery shopping, while we were driving home, we got a call that one of the kid's friends David had committed suicide and another boy was shot and critically injured. This boy turned out to be Tommy. He passed away the next morning from his injury. It was a devastating loss to my children, and to me. We attended his funeral the following week and have been trying to put some order to how one child can kill another and then take his own life. During all of this I felt that I needed to be with my kids more than I needed to go to North Point. In feeling this way, I also felt that I was neglecting mom. I have more than my share of the guilt's.

I think that is what is so difficult for anyone that has a loved one in a nursing home or long-term care facility. You want to be with them, you want them to get better, and you want to be there anytime day or night. The reality is that you still have a life of your own. You still have your good days and bad days. There are bills to pay, children to care for, a house to clean, and your own tragedies as well. It is almost impossible to know when you are visiting enough or when you need to let go of them for a little while and tend your own garden so to speak. If you do not tend what is yours it can get out of control and weeds of separation will grow. If you do not visit, you feel like the worst possible child that ever existed. It is basically a no win situation. The best you can do is try to get through it day by day making the decisions that need to be made for that day and hope that they are the right ones.

I do not have all the answers. Most days I do well to know the question. I just try to spread myself around so that no one falls through the cracks. Ron and the kids are what keep me going.

When Ron started this book, I knew he could say all the " right" words. That is just one of his many talents. He could tell our story, get people to feel what we have gone through, and perhaps touch someone's life that is going through this as well. He could bring them a few laughs and a few tears along the way, but most important to let them know they are not alone in this. He can do all of that. This part of the story he could not tell. He does not have the history or the memories.

I really am writing this for me. I want mom to be real to anyone that reads this. I do not want her to be just a statistic. In a very real sense, writing this is helping me to heal old wounds and helping to form scars finally after all of this time. I guess that is my goal, to tell mom's story, the good and the bad, so that anyone reading this will know there is hope of healing and sometimes just putting it down on paper is an act of helping yourself heal.

Well, I am going to bed now. I am sure there will be things I need to do tomorrow but I made it through another day. I am still happy. I am still very much in love. I am still a mother of four beautiful children. In addition, I am the daughter of an extraordinary woman. I am still here.

Tammy

Update:

It has been three years since the last entry into this journal. We have brought Mary, Carol's mom to Lexington. She is a patient at Northpoint as well. Carol does not really know who she is.

Carol has moved into stage three. She knows Tammy is important to her, but doesn't always make the connection as to whom she actually is. She still remembers me.

Her health is good. Mary is doing well at the moment. Carol is 75. Mary is 94. Jim passed away in April 2007.

We bought a house and moved about 30 miles from Lexington. This makes visits more difficult and less frequent. We are on a waiting list to get Carol moved to a nursing home in our new location. The nursing home is less than five minutes from our home. The delusion that we could care for Carol on our own is completely gone. Both Tammy and I are working outside the home. The two youngest kids are still at home. They are sixteen and eleven now.

There are days we still feel like we are the worst children to ever live for not being able to take care of Carol. Most days, however, we know we are doing what is best for her and Mary.

Tammy's oldest daughter, Sierra, has just had a baby girl, Cloe. Carol will love her. It will be sad, because Carol will love her just as everyone loves a newborn baby. She won't ever know that this wonderful, beautiful bundle of joy is her great granddaughter. She will never realize that part of the mix that makes Cloe so beautiful, includes her. When we tell her Cloe is her great granddaughter, she will be excited. Her excitement will be based on her reaction to our excitement and no recognition of what great granddaughter means. She will see our sadness, even though we try to hide it, and she will feel the pangs of sadness. Even these feelings will be a mystery to her.

Alzheimer's is the great thief. It has taken Carol away from us and left us the empty frame to remind us where she used to be. In this, it is insidious. Sadder still, is that while most patients forget their loved ones, eventually the loved ones forget as well. These pages will assure that Carol will be alive and remembered by someone, beyond tomorrow, long after she has forgotten.

Ron
August 2007

Here is a list of phone numbers we have called in our efforts:

543-0824 ~ The Breckenridge (Private Pay)

246-7000 ~ Eastern State Mental Hospital

246-7452 ~ Randy Moeler (social worker)

800-200-3633 ~ Legal Helpline For OlderKentuckians ~
David Gottfried

245-7136 ~ Adult Protective Services

Mac Colliver (245-5414)

323-5000 ~ UK Medical Center

323-6040 ~ UK Center On Aging

253-3497 ~ Wayne Cook, Asst D.A.

245-5748 ~ Guardianship Services

252-2371 ~ Health Dept

266-5283 ~ Alzheimer's Organization (Corner of High and Euclid
(Fox 56 Building))

269-2325 ~ Ridge Behavioral Health

246-2236 ~ Mental Health Division County Clerks Office
(Fayette)

321-617-7510 ~ Florida State Attorney's office

321-952-4604 ~ Brevard Co. Clerk of the Court

321-617-7284 ~ Judge Turner's office

321-617-7278 (fax)

271-9000 ~ Sayre Christian Village Nursing Home

885-4171 ~ Royal Manor Health Care

(Nicholasville) Susan ~

299-2836 ~ Rose Manor (Melissa Morris)

252-3558 ~ Lexington Center for Health & Rehabilitation (Sherry)

885-3821 ~ Rose Terrace (Rebecca/Jennifer)

252-0871 ~ Homestead Nursing Home (Janet McRobert)
389-9571 (fax)

246-7426 ~ Melissa Pierce (Social Worker ESMH)

502-582-6304 ~ Sen. McConnell's office

502-564-7130 ~ Division of Health & Human Services ~
Dana Abbott

502-564-2474 ~ Kentucky Guardianship Services

502-564-2800 ~ Office of the Inspector General

859-246-2301 ~ Office of the Inspector General

(Lexington Branch) ~ Connie Payne

Rita Satterly (investigator)

253-0593 ~ Ben Cabway~ Court Appt. Attorney (Legal Aid)

800-372-2988 ~ Protection & Advocacy

255-1074 ~ Faith Pharmacy

272-2273 ~ North Point (Cara)

271-2945 Fax

873-4201 ~ Taylor Manor (Private Pay)

277-9215 ~ Ombudsman Agency

278-6072 ~ Bluegrass Ombudsman Agency

321-632-6300 ~ Rockledge Health and Rehabilitation

321-635-9559 (Fax)

About the Author

I have been writing for most of my life. I cannot remember a time in my life when I was not writing. I still have copies of works going back to 1975. I have around 200 poems, of which a few have been published. This is my first attempt at publishing anything longer than a poem.

I have spent my lifetime learning. I am a perpetual student, although not always by choice. I worked 28 years as an Electrician, while also being a minister and Assistant Pastor of a church in that period. That was a constant study, improve, and share cycle. I am now a teacher at a Technology Center for high school students. I am currently in college, after a 30-year absence, to improve on my ability to accomplish this profession. Learning and sharing knowledge has been the one constant in my life. This is just an extension of that.

This journey has been one of learning. This book is my act of sharing it.

www.ingramcontent.com/pod-product-compliance
Lightning Source LLC
Chambersburg PA
CBHW020240290526
45784CB00003B/1047